NEURODEVELOPMENTAL DISEASES - LABORATORY AND CLINICAL RESEARCH

ADHD

COGNITIVE SYMPTOMS, GENETICS AND TREATMENT OUTCOMES

NEURODEVELOPMENTAL DISEASES - LABORATORY AND CLINICAL RESEARCH

Additional books in this series can be found on Nova's website under the Series tab.

Additional e-books in this series can be found on Nova's website under the e-book tab.

NEUROLOGY - LABORATORY AND CLINICAL RESEARCH DEVELOPMENTS

Additional books in this series can be found on Nova's website under the Series tab.

Additional e-books in this series can be found on Nova's website under the e-book tab.

NEURODEVELOPMENTAL DISEASES - LABORATORY AND CLINICAL RESEARCH

ADHD

COGNITIVE SYMPTOMS, GENETICS AND TREATMENT OUTCOMES

RUSSELL THOMPSON
AND
NAOMI J. MILLER
EDITORS

NOVA BIOMEDICAL

New York

For permission to use material from this book please contact us:
Telephone 631-231-7269; Fax 631-231-8175
Web Site: http://www.novapublishers.com

NOTICE TO THE READER

Library of Congress Cataloging-in-Publication Data

ISBN: 978-1-62417-107-9

Library of Congress Control Number: 2012949937

Published by Nova Science Publishers, Inc. † New York

CONTENTS

Preface		**vii**
Chapter 1	Functionality of the ADHD Individual: The Disadvantages and Benefits of Stimulant Treatment *Allison C. Maxwell*	**1**
Chapter 2	Family Dynamics, Conversations and Attachment Patterns: The Construction of ADHD *Rudi Dallos, Cordet Smart and Katie Denman*	**35**
Chapter 3	Do Professions Differ in Their Beliefs about the Causes and Treatment of Attention-Deficit Hyperactivity Disorder? *Rachel Dryer, Michael J. Kiernan and Graham A. Tyson*	**61**
Chapter 4	Motor Coordination Dysfunction in ADHD: New Insights from the Classroom to Genetics *Akio Nakai*	**81**
Chapter 5	Importance of Nutrition Optimization in Multimodal Treatment in Children with Attention-Deficit Hyperactivity Disorder *Teodoro Durá-Travé, María Eugenia Yoldi-Petri and Fidel Gallinas-Victoriano*	**105**

Chapter 6 The Relation between Sluggish Cognitive Tempo and ADHD: A Critical Review **121**
Maria Skounti

Index **131**

PREFACE

Attention-deficit hyperactivity disorder (ADHD) is conceptualized as a neurobehavioral condition that is characterized by developmentally inappropriate levels of inattention, impulsivity and motor overactivity. It is estimated to be present in 3-7% of school-aged populations and can result in significant impairment in academic, social and family functioning. In this book, the authors present current research in the study of the cognitive symptoms, genetics and treatment outcomes of ADHD. Topics discussed include the disadvantages and benefits of stimulant treatment; a discussion on whether professions differ in their beliefs about the causes and treatments of ADHD; motor coordination dysfunction in ADHD; nutrition optimization in the multimodal treatment of ADHD; and the relation between sluggish cognitive tempo and ADHD.

Chapter 1 – This chapter focuses on three aspects of functioning of an individual diagnosed with ADHD: (1) the modification of ADHD symptoms by stimulants vs. depressants; (2) the hyper-focused state created by taking stimulants and its effect on an individual's desire to socialize; and (3) the advantages potentially derived from this hyper-focused state.

As ADHD symptoms are thought to be largely influenced by dopamine levels, it is intriguing that although both stimulant medication and alcohol can increase the amount of the neurotransmitter dopamine in an individual's system, one has the effect of reducing ADHD symptoms (stimulants) and the other seemingly increases symptoms (alcohol).

Stimulant drugs can reduce symptoms of ADHD by increasing focus, reducing hyperactivity, and providing impulse control. However, some side-affects may negatively effect functioning, in particular, the individual's desire to function as a social being. Some individuals with ADHD have noticed a decreased desire to interact with others while taking stimulants, instead falling into a hyper-focused state (sometimes referred to as a "zombie" state) where they neglect relationships in place of time "better spent" focusing on the task at hand.

Conversely, this hyper-focused state may provide an advantage to the individual if their attention is focused on positive tasks (e.g. school, sports or work), leading these individuals to flourish in the activities they chose to focus on while in these hyper-focused states, but harming their abilities in activities outside of this focus.

Findings show that although both stimulant and depressant drugs provide an increase in dopamine levels, the reduction in activity in the central nervous system produced by depressants (e.g. alcohol) results in functioning similar to ADHD symptoms. For those with ADHD, these functions are in addition to the symptoms they already display, accounting for an apparent increase in ADHD symptoms. Stimulant drugs however, increase the amount of dopamine without reducing the activity of the central nervous system, this increase in dopamine level can help return an ADHD individual's functioning's to a "normal" level.

Dosage and type of stimulate can affect if the individual goes into hyper-focus. Although hyper-focus may be beneficial in some areas of life, the detrimental effect it may have in the social realm outweighs the benefits. If an individual suffers from this side-effect they can decide to use medication only during times of focus when socialization is not necessary. This, along with behavioural therapy can help individuals overcome this side-effect while still benefiting from the drugs.

Chapter 2 – This chapter offers a detailed case study of one family taken from a wider research programme investigating the role of family conversational and attachment processes in the development and maintenance of problems labelled as ADHD and self-harm. Individual narrative based attachment assessments and a semi – structured family interview were employed and included an exploration of the current and past problems, family identity, management of feelings, and a family sculpt. Analysis drew on conversational analysis (CA) to focus on the processes of meaning construction between family members. It also utilised the structured form of discourse analysis employed in the Adult Attachment Interview to help reveal defensive processes.

The findings suggested that individual attachment strategies both shaped and were in turn in maintained by the family conversational processes. Specific focus was on how the conversation processes could serve to manage significant attachment dilemmas, such as divided loyalties, triangulation and expressions of anger and protest in the child with the ADHD label.

Chapter 3 – Key health organisations in Western countries, such as the National Institute for Health and Clinical Excellence in the United Kingdom, and more recently, the American Academy of Paediatrics in the United States, have advocated multimodal and multidisciplinary approaches to the diagnosis and treatment of Attention-deficit hyperactivity disorder (ADHD). However, despite these clinical best practice guidelines, there is little evidence of a general adoption of interdisciplinary collaboration and practice. One impediment to the implementation of multidisciplinary practice may be the beliefs that different professionals (and professional bodies) hold about the causes and treatment of ADHD. This chapter reviews the results of research that examined the beliefs of professional groups engaged in the diagnosis and treatment of ADHD about (i) the causes of ADHD and (ii) the efficacy of general treatment approaches. Following the review, other possible impediments to the adoption of interdisciplinary collaboration and practice are also discussed.

Chapter 4 – Clinically, children with ADHD often have so-called "clumsiness," which means motor coordination dysfunction, and previous studies showed the high prevalence of comorbidity as 30~50%. This motor coordination problem is applicable to Developmental Coordination Disorder (DCD) in DSM-IV. Indeed, the results from our community-school based study, using the Japanese version of Developmental Coordination Disorder Questionnaire (DCDQ-J) and ADHD-Rating Scale (ADHD-RS-J), showed that all subscales and total scores of the DCDQ-J were significantly associated with the total and each subscales scores of ADHD-RS-J, which suggested that children with poor motor coordination more frequently showed inattention and hyperactivity.

This frequent and specific comorbidity has led to new concepts or terms, such as DAMP (*Deficits in attention, motor control and perception*) syndrome, DCD-Plus, or different subtype of ADHD. A Swedish cohort study showed that 7.4% of all 7 year-old children had ADHD alone, 7.3% had DCD alone, and 6.6% had the DAMP syndrome, including 1.7% with a so-called 'severe' form. They also mentioned that the severe form of DAMP syndrome has also met criteria of the Autism spectrum disorder, including Asperger's syndrome. Lesson from our community-school based survey showed that, in Japan, 4.2% of children had ADHD alone, 3.8% had DCD alone, and 1.3% had the severe form of DAMP syndrome. Vice versa, 24% of children that had ADHD had DCD and 25% of children that had DCD had ADHD. The other way around, not all children with ADHD have motor coordination dysfunction. These facts might be one of the reasons that previous studies, such as SNPs or brain imaging, sometimes failed the constant and robust results, because of their heterogeneous subjects from these aspects.

While the recent brain imaging study revealed that lower rCBF of some brain lesions and different rCBF response to Methylphenidate were found in an ADHD comorbid DCD group compared to ADHD alone, and genome-wide association study suggested that *MAP2K5* and *CHD6*, and some SNPs might be involved in this combination.

New insights on the motor coordination dysfunction in ADHD from the classroom to genetics could lead to the new concept of disorder, and the new evidence-based diagnosis, medication or intervention.

Chapter 5 – *Background.* Multimodal treatment of attention-deficit hyperactivity disorder (ADHD) combines psychosocial intervention with drug therapy, which, generally, involves a long-term administration of stimulant drugs. Methylphenidate has consistent efficacy with respect to the cardinal symptoms of ADHD and its comorbidity, even though there is some controversy concerning the potential negative influence this drug has on the growth in these patients. This study presents an evolutionary analysis of anthropometric variables in a group of patients diagnosed with ADHD in order to determine the repercussion of drug therapy with osmotic release oral system methylphenidate (OROS-methylphenidate) on the weight and height curve of these patients. The consequences of this nutrition optimization are analyzed.

Patients and methods. Clinical records of 187 patients with ADHD under treatment with OROS-methylphenidate during 30 months (first stage) were reviewed. Weight, height and body mass index values at diagnosis (basal) and after 6, 12, 18, 24 and 30 months of treatment were registered. Subsequently, patients followed a nutritional intervention and weight, height and body mass index were prospectively recorded after 36, 42 and 48 months of follow up (second stage).

Results. Mean age at diagnosis was 8.14 ± 1.6 years. Mean dose of OROS-methylphenidate was gradually increased, from 0.89 ± 0.21 mg/kg/day after 6 months of treatment to 1.05 ± 0.2 mg/kg/day after 30 months (first stage), and 1.31± 0.2 mg/kg/day after 48 months of follow up (second stage). Mean weight at diagnosis was lower than expected mean weight for age in 0.697 kg (weight deficit). This difference increased to 4.274 kg (1.43 kg/year) after 30 months of treatment (first stage), subsequently decreased and was 1.588 kg (0.22 kg/year) after 48 months of treatment (second stage). In the same way, mean height values for these patients at diagnosis were lower than expected mean height values for age in 0.42 cm (height deficit). This difference increased to 2.69 cm (0.91 cm/year) after 30 months of treatment (first stage), subsequently decreased and was 0.83 (0.1 cm/year) after 48 months of follow up (second stage).

Conclusions. Daily treatment with OROS-methylphenidate in patients diagnosed with ADHD has a negative impact in anthropometric variables (weight and height), but the application of nutrition optimization strategies allows recovering weight and height deficit. Nutrition education programs should join multimodal treatments in these patients in order to lessen nutritional problems and the consequences that could be derived from treatment with OROS-methylphenidate.

Chapter 6 – Sluggish Cognitive Tempo (SCT) is a cluster of symptoms including drowsiness, daydreaming, physical hypoactivity, lethargy and apathy. The SCT emerged in association with the ADHD-Inattentive (ADHD-I) type as a great percentage of children diagnosed within this subtype, also present SCT symptoms. Although items relevant to SCT were included in the DSM-IV field trials and were found to associate specifically with the inattentive type of ADHD, they were excluded from the final diagnostic criteria, because of their poor negative predictive power. This omission has led to a long- standing dispute regarding the validity of the ADHD-I type and the use of SCT symptoms as a discriminating factor for the ADHD subtypes. A related debate over the classification of the SCT construct has stimulated considerable research. Although, to date, the construct itself has not been adequately defined, many researchers have proposed that the SCT construct may represent a disorder that is a separate form, but highly co-morbid with ADHD. Additionally, it remains unclear, to what extent the SCT construct is clinically and diagnostically meaningful. The purpose of the present critical review is to analyze the complex relation between ADHD and SCT in terms of diagnostic classification, impairment and comorbidity and to provide future research directions.

In: ADHD
Editors: R. Thompson and N. J. Miller ISBN: 978-1-62417-107-9

Chapter 1

FUNCTIONALITY OF THE ADHD INDIVIDUAL: THE DISADVANTAGES AND BENEFITS OF STIMULANT TREATMENT

Allison C. Maxwell
Carleton University, Ottawa, Ontario, Canada

ABSTRACT

This chapter focuses on three aspects of functioning of an individual diagnosed with ADHD: (1) the modification of ADHD symptoms by stimulants vs. depressants; (2) the hyper-focused state created by taking stimulants and its effect on an individual's desire to socialize; and (3) the advantages potentially derived from this hyper-focused state.

As ADHD symptoms are thought to be largely influenced by dopamine levels, it is intriguing that although both stimulant medication and alcohol can increase the amount of the neurotransmitter dopamine in an individual's system, one has the effect of reducing ADHD symptoms (stimulants) and the other seemingly increases symptoms (alcohol).

Stimulant drugs can reduce symptoms of ADHD by increasing focus, reducing hyperactivity, and providing impulse control. However, some side-affects may negatively effect functioning, in particular, the individual's desire to function as a social being. Some individuals with ADHD have noticed a decreased desire to interact with others while taking stimulants, instead falling into a hyper-focused state (sometimes referred to as a "zombie" state) where they neglect relationships in place of time "better spent" focusing on the task at hand.

Conversely, this hyper-focused state may provide an advantage to the individual if their attention is focused on positive tasks (e.g. school, sports or work), leading these individuals to flourish in the activities they chose to focus on while in these hyper-focused states, but harming their abilities in activities outside of this focus.

Findings show that although both stimulant and depressant drugs provide an increase in dopamine levels, the reduction in activity in the central nervous system produced by depressants (e.g. alcohol) results in functioning similar to ADHD symptoms. For those with ADHD, these functions are in addition to the symptoms they already display, accounting for an apparent increase in ADHD symptoms. Stimulant drugs however, increase the amount of dopamine without reducing the activity of the central nervous system, this increase in dopamine level can help return an ADHD individual's functioning's to a "normal" level.

Dosage and type of stimulate can affect if the individual goes into hyper-focus. Although hyper-focus may be beneficial in some areas of life, the detrimental effect it may have in the social realm outweighs the benefits. If an individual suffers from this side-effect they can decide to use medication only during times of focus when socialization is not necessary. This, along with behavioural therapy can help individuals overcome this side-effect while still benefiting from the drugs.

INTRODUCTION

Attention Deficit Hyperactivity Disorder has quite the history within North America. ADHD, as it is more commonly referred to, was added to the North American manual on the classification of mental disorders, the Diagnostic Statistical Manual (DSM), in 1980 in the DSM-III [Feingold, 2008] and like many other disorders, its symptoms and diagnostic criteria are still being revised. Currently, proposed revisions to the DSM-IV are being reviewed in preparation for the release of its latest version, the DSM-V. According to the American Psychiatric Association's (APA) site for the DSM-V Development [American Psychiatric Association, 2012] this latest version proposes seven adjustments to the section on ADHD (along with rationale for each change); the following changes were taken directly from the APA's DSM-V Development site [American Psychiatric Association, 2012]:

1. Change the age of onset from onset of impairing symptoms by age 7 to onset of symptoms by age 12,
2. Change the three subtypes to three current presentations.
3. Add a fourth presentation for restrictive inattentive;
4. Change the examples in the items, without changing the exact wording of the DSM-IV items, to accommodate a lifespan relevance of each symptom and to improve clarity.
5. Remove PDD from the exclusion criteria.
6. Modify the pre-amble A1 and A2 to indicate that information must be obtained from two different informants (parents and teachers for children and third party/significant other for adults) whenever possible.
7. Still under consideration: Adjust the cut point for diagnosis in adults.

These proposals reflect an ever changing mind-set about this disorder. Over the years since ADHD surfaced, there has been an increase in diagnoses as the disorder has become more well-known, indeed, parents, teachers and even friends and co-workers have begun to identify the signs of ADHD within individuals they know. With this increase of identification have come changes to the way we view this disorder. Originally, ADHD was viewed as a childhood disorder that was primarily found in young boys. Now, as reflected in the changes to the DSM-V, we have come to realize that ADHD can be identified in the adult population (adult ADHD). In addition to the changes in identifying individuals with ADHD, have come changes in the prescribed treatment of individuals diagnosed with ADHD. In 1937 Charles Bradley discovered that stimulant medication was capable of reducing symptoms of ADHD in individuals [Hallowell and Ratey, 1994; Hoffman, 2004]. In response to this discovery, drug companies developed various prescription stimulant medications to aid in the reduction of ADHD symptoms. However, these medication have often come at the price of side-effects such as irritability, addiction, "zombie-like" states and reduced desire to socialize, headaches, stomachaches, loss of appetite, increased blood pressure, sadness, anxiety, etc. [Breggin, 1998; Davis-Berman, and Pestello, 2010; Doggett, 2004; Pearson, Santos, Roache, Casat, Loveland, Lachar, Lane, Faria, and Cleveland, 2003; Smith, Pelham, Evans, Gnagy, Molina, Bukstein, Greiner, Myak, Presnell, and Willoughby, 1998]. In addition, students at colleges and universities became aware of the increased focus achievable through the use of these prescription drugs and started taking them in order to focus while studying for exams in the hopes of increasing their performance. In response to these negative effects of medication, individuals started promoting instead, cognitive behavioural therapy, educational intervention, electro-encephalograph neurofeedback, diet, social skills training, parent training, education regarding ADHD, and various forms of behaviour therapy (designed to reinforce attentive, goal-directed behaviours while reducing or ridding the individual of impulsive, hyperactive behaviours) [Centers for Disease Control and Prevention, 2009; Children and Adults with Attention-Deficit-/Hyperactivity Disorder (CHADD), 2012; Doggett, 2004]. These treatments result in fewer side-effects and can be highly effective in treating ADHD symptoms. Although these treatments and many others are still being used, a combined form of medication and behavioural therapy (multimodal) is promoted by many to be the best approach [Centers for Disease Control and Prevention, 2009; Conners, et al., 2001; Doggett, 2004].

This author intends to expand on the topics covered in this brief review of ADHD. In particular, this chapter will begin by outlining some facts about how we diagnosis and identify individuals with ADHD, how the number of individuals diagnosed as ADHD has grown recently and why this may be, as well as a brief description of treatments other than stimulant medication used to treat those with ADHD. Finally, the author will turn to the main focus of this chapter which intends to cover the following three topics of interest that arise from the above brief review of ADHD and its treatment methods:

1. The author intends to explore the seemingly paradoxical treatment method of stimulant drugs, specifically, why ADHD symptoms appear to diminish with the consumption of stimulant medication (e.g. methylphenidate such as Ritalin or amphetamine such as Adderal), but appear to increase with the consumption of depressants such as alcohol.
2. Second, the author intends to focus on a particular side-effect of stimulant medications: the "zombie effect"/reduced desire to socialize. Stimulant drugs claim to reduce inattentiveness of individuals with ADHD by providing them with the ability to focus on mundane tasks that they would otherwise be distracted from. However, this ability to focus on a task may drive the individual into a hyper-focused state, reducing an individual's desire to pull focus away and socialize. Indeed, some individuals have noticed a decreased desire to interact with others while taking prescription stimulants; neglecting relationships in place of time "better spent" focusing on the task at hand.

3. Finally, it is with curiosity that the author approaches the topic of possible benefits derived from this hyper-focused state. It is arguable that this ability to focus on mundane tasks may lead an individual to obtain higher level careers or achieve a higher education…even if it is at the expense of neglecting social responsibilities. However, it is possible, that the benefits derived from stimulant medication may still be obtained by individuals if they use a more even distribution of drug therapy and behaviour therapy. It is the opinion of this researcher that using a combination of drugs and behavioural therapy could provide the individuals with the focus they need to perform well in school and work situations, while using behavioural therapy in place of the drug could allow the individual to keep their desire to socialize and also provide them with the skills necessary to do so.

About ADHD: The Facts

How Do We Identify and Diagnosis ADHD?

Attention Deficit Hyperactivity Disorder, or ADHD (the same as Attention Deficit Disorder, with the addition of a hyperactive state) is a disorder characterized by inattention, impulsivity and hyperactivity. It is a recognized and treated disorder in many parts of the world, although it is most widely recognized and treated in North America and the United Kingdom (in the UK, hyperkinetic disorder is the official term used) [Singh, 2008]. North America uses the Diagnostic and Statistical Manual (DSM) in order to diagnose individuals with ADHD while the UK uses the International Statistical Classification of Diseases and Related Health Problems, more commonly referred to as the ICD (International Classification of Diseases). As this chapter is primarily focused on North American research, the DSM will be used. The DSM-V is currently in its final stages of revision before release; since it has not yet been finalized, the fourth edition, which is still in use, will be referred to throughout this chapter.

Professionals refer to the DSM in order to rate an individual on symptoms pertaining to ADHD. An individual may be classified as either: (1) ADHD, predominately inattentive type; (2) ADHD, predominately hyperactive-impulsive type; or (3) ADHD, combined type (if both other sub-type criteria are met). Although some behavioural tendencies are almost always seen in individuals diagnosed with ADHD, not every individual will show the same characteristics and likewise, not every individual will display these behaviours at the same level of severity. Although the DSM does not identify this behavioural spectrum specifically, it does note that only a certain amount of criteria is necessary to diagnosis an individual with ADHD, and therefore, professionals realize that the amount of criteria that fit the individual may lead to identifying how severely the symptoms may affect the individual in their daily life. These criteria, along with accounts from others of the individual's behavioural tendencies, can lead professionals to make appropriate assessments of the individual and also guide them to administer an appropriate level of treatment.

Researchers of the paper "The Clinically Meaningful Link Between Alcohol Use and Attention Deficit Hyperactivity Disorder" [Smith, Brooke, and Pelham, 2002], provide a comprehensive report of the diagnostic criteria for identifying ADHD outlined in the DSM-IV. It is displayed below:

In order to be diagnosed with ADHD, a person must meet the criteria for one of the three subtypes of ADHD (predominately inattentive type, predominately hyperactive/impulsive type, or combined type). In addition, they must:

- Have symptoms that have persisted for at least 6 months and which must be present to a degree that creates problems and is inconsistent with developmental level.
- Have at least one symptom that caused impairment before the age of 7.
- Have some symptoms that are present in at least two different settings (e.g., home, school), and that cause clinically significant impairment in social or academic functioning.
- Have symptoms that are not associated with another disorder (e.g., psychotic disorder, mood disorder, personality disorder, or anxiety disorder).

1. Predominately Inattentive Type: Six symptoms of inattention, as listed below

- Fails to give close attention to details or makes careless mistakes
- Has difficultly sustaining attention in tasks or play activities.
- Does not seem to listen when spoken to directly.

- Does not follow through on instructions and fails to finish tasks (not as a result of oppositional behaviour or failure to understand instructions).
- Has difficulties organizing tasks and activities.
- Avoids or dislikes tasks that require sustained mental effort.
- Loses things necessary for tasks or activities (e.g., toys, books).
- Is easily distracted.
- Is forgetful in daily activities.

2. Predominately Hyperactive/Impulsive Type: Six symptoms of hyperactivity/impulsivity, as listed below

- Fidgets with hands or feet or squirms in seat
- Leaves seat in classroom or in other situations in which remaining seated as expected.
- Runs or climbs excessively when it is inappropriate.
- Has difficulty playing or engaging in leisure activities quietly.
- Is always "on the go" or acts as if "driven by a motor".
- Talks excessively.
- Blurts out answers before questions have been complete.
- Has difficulty awaiting their turn.
- Interrupts or intrudes on others (e.g., interrupts conversations or games).

3. Combined type: Six Symptoms from each of the previous lists

Prevalence of the Disorder in North American Society Today

Chances are, in your lifetime you have come in contact with at least one individual who has been diagnosed, or will be diagnosed, with ADHD. In fact, with the growing number of individuals being classified as ADHD, it would not be surprising if you are related to, work closely with, or have a close personal relationship with someone with this disorder. This is so likely because according to recent studies on the topic, ADHD is the most common childhood neurobehavioural disorder [Visser, Bitsko, Danielson, Perou, and Blumberg, 2010]. According to an article posted by the Centers for Disease Control and Prevention on November 12, 2010, [Visser, Bitsko, Danielson,

Perou, and Blumberg, 2010] the National Survey of Children's health reported in 2007 that the number of children ages 4-17 who have ever received a diagnose of ADHD had increased from 7.8% to 9.5% during 2003-2007; this meant that in just 4 years ADHD diagnoses had increased by 21.8%. In another study recounted by an article on Psych Central [Nauert, 2012] researchers reported that from 2000 to 2010 the rate of ADHD diagnosis was up by 66 percent. In addition to this increase in diagnosis of children with ADHD, we now recognize that individuals can carry ADHD symptoms into adulthood [Faraone, and Biederman, 2005]. This realization is reflected in the changes to the diagnostic criteria in the DSM [American Psychiatric Association, 2012]. With these drastic increases and expansion of the diagnostic criteria for ADHD (now including adults), questions have begun to surface regarding the legitimacy of diagnoses – individuals have begun to wonder if those being diagnosed with ADHD truly carry the characteristics of ADHD, or if we are beginning to over-use and abuse the behavioural characteristics attributed to it in order to diagnose stressful life in adulthood and normal rambunctious childhood behaviour.

Over-Diagnosis and Over-Medication?

In their book "Selling Sickness", Ray Moynihan and Alan Cassels [2005] take the position that the drug companies which develop/sell the prescription medications used to treat disorders such as ADHD are in large part, the reason why there has been an increase in the number of individuals being diagnosed with the disorder. The authors seem to argue that although these symptoms of ADHD (impulsivity, hyperactivity, lack of focus, etc.) may arise in some individuals, we have been bombarded with propaganda through advertisements and awareness campaigns and even broadened the definition of ADHD so that more and more people feel as though they or someone they know fit the diagnostic criteria for the disorder.

To a degree, it is hard to argue that this is not the case, if an individual is unfocused or hyperactive, many will jokingly comment that they probably have ADHD. Even on popular television shows we see recants of individuals with such behavioural problems. For example, the Simpsons, in season 11 show an episode titled "Brother's Little Helper" where the character Bart Simpson, is diagnosed with ADD and put on a drug called "Focusyn" to help him with the disorder. Also, on the newly popular show Modern Family, in episode 8 of their first season titled "Starry Night" we see one of the family members (Alex Dunphy) arguing that her brother (Luke Dunphy) has ADHD. As Alex recites the symptoms of ADHD we see examples of how the father (Phil Dunphy) displays these same symptoms.

It is certain that our society is more aware of ADHD and ADD and the symptoms associated with it, but with this increased awareness sometimes comes the over diagnosis and exaggeration of symptoms. Dr. Lawrence Diller, in "Selling Sickness" [Moynihan, and Cassels, 2005] argues that we seem to be beginning to medicate childhood behaviours, not just full-blown ADHD behaviours. Diller observes that the patients he was seeing coming to his office were not necessarily showing very strong symptoms of ADHD, instead they may show subtle symptoms of ADHD but really, the only issue was that they or their parents/guardians thought they were not doing as well in school as they should be doing [Moynihan, and Cassels, 2005]. Diller goes on to say "I began to wonder if boyhood, at least in my community, has become a disease." Of course now, as noted above, we are no longer simply focusing on the fidgety child unable to concentrate in a classroom for extended periods of time, now there is also a push to diagnose and medicate adults with ADHD. In adulthood however the marketing campaigns are targeting what appears to be a stressful work life, which certainly, the majority of individuals can relate to. This ad from Lilly (a leading prescription drug company) in particular was quoted by Moynihan and Cassels [2005]:

> "Distracted? Disorganized? Frustrated? Modern Life or Adult ADD? Many adults have been living with Adult attention deficit disorder (Adult ADD) and don't recognize it. Why? Because its symptoms are often mistaken for stressful life." [Moynihan and Cassels, 2005]

According to one marketing professional, Vince Parry, noted in "Selling Sickness" [Moynihan, and Cassels, 2005], the way these drugs are being marketed to people is by telling us the behaviours we see every day in ourselves are not normal, but in fact are part of a new condition we never realized we had before: "It's raising the level of awareness about something we don't even know we have until we began looking into this further" [Moynihan, and Cassels, 2005].

So, is it possible that the arguments made by Moynihan and Cassels and other authors with them [Breggin, 2001; Davis-Berman, and Pestello, 2010] are true? Could we be over-diagnosing and over-medicating individuals who do not actually have ADHD? It is possible. However, this increase in diagnosis may simply be a result of increased awareness of a problem that people didn't realize they could solve before. Individuals do suffer from the inability to focus, inattention and hyperactivity that make their lives difficult. Who are we to claim that they do not have these symptoms and that they are not debilitating to their lifestyles? The fact is, there are individuals suffering from the symptoms outlined in the DSM-IV for ADHD and they are benefiting from stimulant medications. There will always be problems with the diagnosis of a disease we cannot physically see the characteristics of, but only the individual can tell if they are truly there. All we can do is take every precaution to ensure that individuals are not being over-diagnosed and that newly found information is included in our diagnosis. This is being done with the revisions of the DSM [American Psychiatric Association, 2012].

What Are the Treatments for ADHD?

In 1985, researchers, Rapport, Stoner, DuPaul, Birmingham, and Tucker identified psychostimulant medications (e.g. methylphenidate) as the most commonly used treatment for individuals diagnosed with ADHD. They attributed this popularity with the many behavioural benefits cited by research papers before them.

These benefits included: providing the individuals with shot-term sustained attention, lowered activity level, better academic performance, reduced impulsivity and improved classroom decorum. According to researchers from a paper published in 1991 [Whalen, and Henker, 1991], 60% to 90% of children diagnosed with ADHD were using stimulant medication for prolonged periods in order to treat their symptoms.

Individuals with ADHD who use stimulant medication do often find improvements in their symptoms and for this reason medication is still a prominent method of treatment for individuals with ADHD. However, stimulant medications are by no means the only treatment prescribed by professionals. Indeed, more recently professionals and awareness groups have begun to promote a multimodal approach to treating individuals with ADHD [Centers for Disease Control and Prevention, 2009; Conners, et al., 2001; Doggett, 2004] and some argue stimulant medication should only be used as a complementary treatment method if necessary [Whalen, and Henker, 1991].

Researchers have discovered that not only are there non-stimulant medications that can be used for individuals with ADHD, but that medications in general are not the only way that individuals with ADHD can combat symptoms. Other methods work well for individuals with ADHD, such as cognitive behavioural therapy, educational intervention, electroencephalograph neurofeedback, diet, social skills training, parent training, education regarding ADHD, etc. [Centers for Disease Control and Prevention, 2009; Children and Adults with Attention-Deficit/Hyperactivity Disorder (CHADD), 2012; Doggett, 2004]. Intensive summer treatment programs, such as the one mentioned by Smith et al. [1998] in their study, have also been a popular method of providing treatment for individuals with ADHD [Kail, and Barnfield, 2009].

According to CHADD, a well known organization that provides information and support to parents, professionals and individuals with ADD and ADHD, effective treatment for children and teens with ADHD requires a combination of parent training, behavioural interventions, educational programming, education regarding ADHD and, if necessary, medication. On the CHADD website, it is noted that adults with ADHD benefit most from a team approach (which could include healthcare professionals, significant others, family members, etc.).

This team, along with the individual work together in providing a structured environment, vocational counseling and psychotherapy for the individual. Adults may also benefit from medication, but it is not noted as the primary focus for treatment [Children and Adults with Attention-Deficit/Hyperactivity Disorder (CHADD), 2012].

It is likely that medication is being phased out as a treatment for individuals with ADHD, not only because these medications are sometimes attributed with negative side-effects, but also because the skills that individuals with ADHD lack (e.g. control, focus, attention, scalability) are not developed by using these medications. Indeed, according to Whalen and Henker [1991] "non-pharmacologic treatments focused on building social repertoires and mastering self-regulation are needed to help youngsters with ADHD catch up to their peers in the interpersonal domain." In particular, therapy focuses on reinforcing positive behaviour while teaching the individual to inhibit negative behaviour (e.g. impulsivity and hyperactivity) [Kail, and Barnfield, 2009]. Although it will be quite some time before we see a very large flux away from the use of stimulant medication to treat individuals with ADHD, it is the hope of this researcher, and of many others, that this increase in alternative methods of treating individuals with ADHD (especially behavioural therapy) will provide these individuals with more positive skills, less negative side-effects and a decreased dependence on medication in their daily lives.

Summary and Introduction to the Three Main Topics

Now that we have covered how ADHD is identified and diagnosed, what the prevalence of this disorder is, and how professionals go about treating individuals with it, we can turn to the main topic of this chapter: the effects of stimulant treatment on the functionality of the ADHD individual. Three subtopics will be the base of this assessment: (1) why are stimulant medications used to treat individuals diagnosed as hyperactive? (2) What are the possible side-effects of using stimulant medication (in particular, how do these side-effects affect the individuals in regards to socializing?) (3) Does stimulant medication provide the individual with an unfair advantage above their peers?

TOPIC #1: TREATMENT – WHY ARE STIMULANTS USED TO TREAT INDIVIDUALS DIAGNOSED AS HYPERACTIVE?

Discovery of the Use of Stimulants as a Treatment for Hyperactive Children

Although it is hard to pin-point an exact date when ADHD was first identified, many will agree that the first documented evidence of ADHD symptoms actually appeared in a poem written by Heinrich Hoffmann in 1845. This poem was titled "The Story of Fidgety Philip"; it was part of a book of children's poetry Hoffmann wrote on children's behaviours in order to amuse his son [Feingold, 2008]. The poem outlines some of the common symptoms found in today's definition of ADHD such as hyperactivity, restlessness, impulsivity and inattention. A copy of the English translation of this poem appears below [Hoffman, 2004]:

The Story of Fidgety Philip
"Let me see if Philip can
Be a little gentleman;
Let me see if he is able
To sit still for once at table":
Thus Papa bade Phil behave;
And Mamma looked very grave.
But fidgety Phil,
He won't sit still;

He wriggles,
And giggles,
And then, I declare,
Swings backwards and forwards,
And tilts up his chair,
Just like any rocking horse –
"Philip! I am getting cross!"

See the naughty, restless child
Growing still more rude and wild,
Till his chair falls over quite.
Philip screams with all his might,
Catches at the cloth, but then
That makes matters worse again.
Down upon the ground they fall,
Glasses, plates, knives, forks, and all.
How Mamma did fret and frown,
When she saw them tumbling down!
And Papa made such a face!
Philip is in sad disgrace.

Where is Philip, where is he?
Fairly covered up you see!
Cloth and all are lying on him;
He has pulled down all upon him.
What a terrible to-do!
Dishes, glasses, snapt in two!
Here a knife, and there a fork!
Philip, this is cruel work.
Table all so bare, and ah!
Poor Papa, and poor Mamma
Look quite cross, and wonder how
They shall have their dinner now.

In 1902, over 50 years after Hoffmann wrote this poem, a paediatrician named George Still, provided more detail on a condition where individuals displayed symptoms similar to those now associated with ADHD [Feingold, 2008]. Still's recant of this condition is said to be an expression of a group of children he had studied who displayed signs of defiance, excessive emotionality, passion, lawlessness, spitefulness, and who displayed little inhibitory volition [Hallowell, and Ratey, 1994]. Still believed that these symptoms were not simply the result of neglectful parents who did not foster appropriate behaviours in their children, nor did he believe situational factors were to blame, instead, Still attributed these behaviours to genetics, stating that they were hereditary [Hallowell, and Ratey, 1994].

William James later posited that individuals who displayed a lack of inhibition, moral control and sustained attention may not have the same ability to inhibit their reactions to stimuli as others. More specifically, he suggested that a malfunction in the brain may be the case of this reduced ability, resulting in the problematic behaviour displayed [Hallowell, and Ratey, 1994]. This theory paved the road for Eugene Kahn and Louis H. Cohen, who in 1934 published a paper on a theory they called "Organic Driveness". In their research they argued that biology was to blame for this behavioural disorder where individuals displayed hyperactivity, impulsiveness, and moral immaturity. In their paper they argued that symptoms such as impaired attention, regulation of activity and impaired impulse control were displayed by those who had been affected by the encephalitis epidemic. As this epidemic affected neurological functions, it followed that individuals displaying these symptoms may also have affected neurological functions; this meant that the problem may be attributed to disease, not to heredity [Feingold, 2008; Hallowell, and Ratey, 1994]. Not long after the publication of this research in 1937, Charles Bradley was credited with the discovery of using stimulant medications (at the time, using Benzedrine) to treat individuals with these behavioural tendencies. Although it still seems counterintuitive to use a stimulant medication in order to reduce the activities of a hyperactive individual, this medication seemed to work, and is still primarily used for the treatment of ADHD symptoms today [Feingold, 2008; Hallowell, and Ratey, 1994].

How Do Stimulants Work to Reduce Symptoms of ADHD?

So, why did Bradley's use of stimulant medication work to reduce symptoms in hyperactive children? To answer this we might want to touch on the theory put forth by Maurice Laufer in 1957 which stated that a malfunction in the thalamus (the part of the brain responsible for sensory perception and regulation as well as motor function) reduced the individual's ability to filter stimuli appropriately, so, those with the malfunction suffered from an overload of stimuli and in turn hyperactivity of this part of the brain [Hallowell, and Ratey, 1994]. Another brain-based hypothesis came about later in 1970 when C. Kornetsky developed the "Catecholamine Hypothesis of Hyperactivity" which stated that there is an underproduction or underutilization of the neurotransmitters norepinephrine and dopamine in the brain [Hallowell, and Ratey, 1994].

Combined with what we know today about the brain's functioning, these theories have provided us with a foundation for discerning why Bradley's use of stimulants worked to reduce the symptoms displayed by individuals with ADHD.

We now know that the brain functions through the production, release and uptake of neurotransmitters. Neurotransmitters can be thought of as internal communication signals used within the brain to communicate between its various parts. Communication occurs between neurons when one neuron produces a neurotransmitter and then releases it (this neuron is called the presynaptic neuron) into the open space (called a synapse) between another neuron (known as the postsynaptic neuron), the postsynaptic neuron then absorbs the neurotransmitter and the signal is passed down the line until the communication is received by the targeted area and the appropriate function is carried out. When neurotransmitters are released into the synapse not all bind to the postsynaptic neuron, those that do not bind are reabsorbed by the presynaptic neuron (a process referred to as reuptake). A problem occurs in individuals with ADHD where there is either not enough of the neurotransmitter dopamine or norepinephrine produced or it is reabsorbed too quickly, this results in the message(s) not being sent or received in sufficient time [Low, 2010].

Stimulants such as methylphenidate (more commonly known as Ritalin, Metadate and Concerta) and amphetamines (more commonly known as Dexedrine and Adderall) are used to regulate this communication problem by blocking or slowing down the reuptake of these neurotransmitters (the primary function of methylphenidate) or by producing more of them (the primary function of amphetamines), allowing more time for the postsynaptic neuron to effectively receive and pass along the message. The appropriate production and usage of these neurotransmitters is important in the ability of the brain to regulate attention and executive function (e.g. the ability to organize and manage tasks) [Low, 2010].

Stimulants help to focus an individual's attention on the task at hand. For those with ADHD, being able to focus is hard and being able to focus on just one task or on a very mundane task is extremely difficult. Taking stimulant medication can therefore help these individuals improve their focus by managing incoming stimuli appropriately; this allows them to perform better on tasks where sustained attention is necessary. Unfortunately, these drugs do not help an individual evaluate a stimulus in order to choose an appropriate reaction; rather, they just limit output responses [Advokat, 2010]. This means that for instance, in social situations, individuals with ADHD who take stimulant medication will be less likely to blurt out inappropriately or become distracted or lose track of a conversation, but it does not mean they will be better at the actual interaction. Learning appropriate social skills usually comes from observing others socializing and noting what is deemed appropriate and not appropriate in turn. Individuals with ADHD are recorded as observing social interactions of their peers less and are generally noted as having more difficulty acting appropriately in social situations than their peers without ADHD [Whalen, and Henker, 1991]. Therefore, even though individuals with ADHD may seem to act more appropriately in social situations because while on medication they are less likely to become distracted or speak out unnecessarily, they may still lack the social skills generally developed through observation. This is often why behavioural therapy is useful for individuals with ADHD: it can be used to help them develop and understand appropriate social skills [Whalen, and Henker, 1991].

Why Are Depressants Not Used to Treat Individuals with ADHD?

Although it may have at first seemed contradictory to use a stimulant to reduce the undesirable behaviours in a hyperactive individual, this approach worked and when reviewed, as we have done above, it is obvious why this method works. Depressants, on the other hand, may seem more appropriate in reducing symptoms of ADHD in individuals as it is a kind of sedative, however, research has found that depressants do not reduce the symptoms of ADHD and in fact, they may even aggravate these symptoms. Why might that be? To find out, we must first understand how depressants function.

Depressants, like stimulants, affect neurotransmitter activity, particularly the activity of the neurotrsamitter GABA (gamma-aminobutyric acid). GABA's function is to produce a calming or sedative effect on the individual. Depressants increase the activity of GABA which results in the dulled reactions seen in individuals taking depressants [Spine Universe, 2010]. Alcohol is a type of non-medicated depressant drug commonly used in social situations. As this author has reported before [Maxwell, 2011] alcohol has a similar effect in the production of dopamine as do prescription stimulant medications. Alcohol both increases the development and decreases the reuptake of the neurotransmitter dopamine in the brain. Although both dopamine and norepinephrine have been attributed to the symptoms displayed by individuals with ADHD, many researchers relate the dopamine system in particular with ADHD symptoms; this theory has been called the "dopaminergic hypothesis" [Prediger, Pamplona, Fernandes, and Takahashi, 2005]. The Dopaminergic hypothesis is basically the same as that which has been outlined above, that production and reuptake of dopamine is affected in individuals with ADHD.

So, since alcohol increases the production of dopamine and also reduces the reuptake of it (effects which are also caused by stimulants), we could expect to see similar results from individuals with ADHD who drink alcohol as we do with individuals with ADHD who take prescription stimulant drugs (e.g. regulated symptoms of ADHD). However, while alcohol provides that boost of dopamine that individuals with ADHD are searching for it also depresses the central nervous system. So, instead of creating the feeling of alertness, control and focus, we see a reduction in inhibitory controls, focus and attention. In other words, even though the depressant may be providing the individual with more signals to the brain (increased production of dopamine) the brain functions have been slowed down by the other chemicals produced by the depressant, offsetting the effects of the increased availability of dopamine.

It is possible that not only do depressants not reduce ADHD symptoms, but they may also *increase* these symptoms while the individual is under the influence. The study performed by Weafer, Fillmore, and Milich [2009] compared the effects of alcohol on participants diagnosed as having ADHD with participants without this diagnosis in order to see if there were differences in their abilities to perform tasks and inhibit incorrect responses to tasks under the influence of alcohol. It was suggested that those with ADHD would show increased sensitivity to inhibitory controls while under the influence of alcohol when compared to those without ADHD [Weafer, Fillmore, and Milich, 2009]. The researchers' results supported this suggestion, showing a higher rate of alcohol impairment in adults with ADHD (e.g. higher rates of impulsive behaviours and lower rates of impulse control) than in adults without this diagnosis. The reason behind these findings is explained in the researchers' hypothesis. This explanation is also shared with the researchers of the article [Smith, Molina, and Pelham, 2002]. They explain that because the symptoms produced by alcohol (such as disturbances in cognitive functioning, inattention, reduced ability to inhibit inappropriate responses, and in some cases hyperactivity) are so similar to those exhibited by individuals with

ADHD, when individuals with ADHD consume alcohol, these symptoms will be exaggerated more than in those without ADHD [Weafer, Fillmore, and Milich, 2009].

Conclusion: Why Stimulants Rather Than Depressants Are Used to Treat Individuals with ADHD

Individuals with ADHD who display signs of *overstimulation* are ironically, suffering from an *under-stimulation* of certain chemicals in the brain necessary to produce functions such as impulse control, focus, attention, etc. Therefore, although it may seem strange to provide stimulants to overactive individuals, these particular drugs are used to stimulate the production of signals to parts of the brain that allow the individual to inhibit hyperactive and impulsive behaviour [Kail, and Barnfield, 2009]. And, unlike depressants, they do not reduce the functioning of other parts of the brain in the process. For this reason, depressants are not used for treating individuals with over stimulation; instead doctors turn to the seemingly paradoxical treatment of stimulant medication.

Topic #2: Effects of Stimulant Drugs, Particularly on Socialization

Stimulant Drug Side-Effects

Although, as noted above, stimulant drugs have historically been the go-to method of treating individuals with ADHD, side-effects have sometimes occurred in individuals taking the medications. These side-effects include stomachaches, headaches, irritability, loss of appetite, reduced desire to socialize, "zombie-like" behaviour, addiction, increased blood pressure, sadness, anxiety, etc. [Breggin, 1998; Davis-Berman, and Pestello, 2010; Doggett, 2004; Pearson, et al., 2003; Smith, et al., 1998]. One may ask then if stimulants may cause side-effects and there are other treatment methods available, why are stimulant medications still being used as the primarily mode of treating individuals with ADHD? The answer is simple, medication is a "quick-fix" compared to options such as behavioural therapy, and modifying an individual's environment to help them control their ADHD symptoms may not be feasible. For instance, restructuring of the classroom or work-place may provide individuals with ADHD a better advantage in these area of their lives, and reduce the negative effects of their symptoms on their work, but unfortunately, our workplace, school systems and even our at home resources are usually very limited. The work environment is structured a particular way to provide fast and effective results to clients, it is not easily changed for one individual who has problems concentrating or working in that kind of environment. Teachers have large classroom sizes and understandably have difficulty dedicating more of their attention to one student or changing their teaching styles to benefit a few out of a group. At the same time, parents/guardians may be working all day and/or busy with other children or engagements and the addition of a hyperactive child may be excessively tiring. So, in the end the draw of a drug that can quickly calm these disruptive behaviours and provide focus to the individual may be very tempting for all involved (individuals with ADHD, co-workers, bosses, teachers and parents alike).

Additionally, like any drug, the side-effects will depend on the individual, the dosage and the drug. As indicated in the section above describing the effects of stimulant medication, not all stimulant drugs act in the same way. For instance, methylphenidate (e.g. Ritalin, Metadate and Concerta) functions to primarily block or slow the reuptake of neurotransmitters, while amphetamines (e.g. Dexedrine and Adderall) primarily produce more neurotransmitters [Low, 2010]. This difference in how these two stimulants affect an individual's dopamine and norepinephrine systems can be one reason why individuals with ADHD react differently to different stimulant medications [Low, 2010]. In terms of side-effects, doctors will generally prescribe a particular drug for one reason or another to an individual with ADHD and assess the positive effects of the drug and any negative side-effects by trying a range of safe dosages. This allows them to find out what dosage and type of drug works best for each individual [Rapport, Stoner, DuPaul, Birmingham, and Tucker, 1985]. Furthermore, most of the side-effects that do arise are relatively minor and can be reduced by reducing the amount of drug, discontinuing use of the drug altogether or switching to a different drug.

How Socialization Is Affected

Although it is true that individuals may be able to observe most side-effects quite easily (e.g. stomachache, headache, lack of appetite, sleep deprivation, etc.), it is possible that one side-effect in particular may go overlooked because its symptoms may seem to be a reduction in ADHD characteristics and therefore a mistaken indication that the drug is working; this side-effect is: decreased desire for socialization. Decreased desire to socialize may go unnoted because it is usually paired with an increased desire to focus on other positive tasks, such as school work [Breggin, 1998; Davis-Berman, and Pestello, 2010]. This increased focus is sometimes referred to as the "zombie-effect". Countless studies focused on obtaining more information on the effects of medications provided to individuals with ADHD have also noted social withdrawal, diminished social interaction or social play, over-focused behaviour or zombie-like behaviours (e.g. the "zombie-effect") [Breggin, 1998; Breggin, 2001; Pearson, et al., 2003; Rapport, Stoner, DuPaul, Birmingham, and Tucker, 1985; Vanderschuren, Trezza, Griffioen-Roose, Schiepers, Van Leeuwen, De Vries, and Schoffelmeer, 2008; Whalen, and Henker, 1991].

Smith, et al. [1998] set out to identify at what dosage level individuals taking methylphenidate recorded the most positive benefits in terms of social behaviour with the least amount of negative side-effects. The researchers described negative social behaviour as "fighting with peers, noncompliance with parental rules or requests, and disruptive behavior in the classroom". Participants of the study were provided with either a placebo or various dosages of methylphenidate (either 10-mg, 20-mg or 30-mg). The results showed improvement in social behaviour at all dosage levels but the authors noted that when individuals showed positive effects at lower dosage levels increasing the dosage generally did not improve social behaviour by much. In addition any dosage higher than 10-mg was usually paired with negative side-effects such as social withdrawal, dulled affect, stomachache, and loss of appetite, noting that social withdrawal began as early as with a dosage of 20-mg and got worse with higher dosage. The authors therefore concluded that as benefits were derived at a lower level of dosage there was no need to risk negative side-effects by increasing the dosage, especially since any increased benefit was so minimal once achieved at the lower levels.

In another study, Davis-Berman, and Pestello [2010] researched the effects of medications on individuals with ADHD and noted similar social withdrawal side-effects in some participants. In this study, the authors explore the social experiences of individuals taking medication for ADD/ADHD through one-on-one interviews using open ended and trigger questions. In terms of desire to socialize, the results showed that the increase in focus the drugs provided was often paired with a decrease in social interests and skills.

> "Personality change was often mentioned as a problem, with respondents saying that by increasing their ability to focus, their social skills and interests decreased. Some said that they felt that their former friendliness was masked due to the medication." [Davis-Berman, and Pestello, 2010]

Individuals were quoted throughout the study identifying the changes in their personalities in general and their desires to socialize in particular. One individual was quoted as saying: "I didn't like the fact that it (medication) made me really quiet. I was talkative and outgoing, and then when I started taking it I was really quiet". Another individual admitted that "when I was on medication for ADD, I didn't want to talk to my friends, I just wanted to do my homework".

This research also documented that individuals would sometimes take what they referred to as "drug holidays", where the individuals would take their medications when at school during the week, but on the weekend they would not take it and the changes in their attitude and behaviour were quite different during these drug holidays compared with when they were taking the drugs. This type of behaviour was also noted in "Selling Sickness" where an individual admitted that his daughter who was taking the drugs would only take them during academic times of need [Moynihan, and Cassels, 2005].

Additionally, there are online forums where individuals with ADHD or individuals who know someone diagnosed with ADHD converse about various topics on the disorder. Individuals on these forums have described changes in their significant others or themselves in terms of socialization while on prescription stimulants. In one forum individuals converse about how Ritalin in particular has affected their social skills; two individuals find that it is causing them to become awkward in conversations, providing them with increased concentration on other things ("important stuff") and not on the socialization going on [WrongPlanet.net, 2011]. In contrast, however, the third individual noted that they found the effects of Ritalin to provide them with an increased ability to focus on conversations. As noted earlier, the effects drugs have on individuals may vary depending on the dosage and the individual themselves. However, it could also be interpretation of the drugs, while two individuals interpret the effects of Ritalin to be negative because they are focusing on other tasks and not on socialization, the third individual interprets the effects as positive because they are focusing on the social situation – all individuals may be hyper-focusing, but the focus of their hyper-focusing could be directed at different things (school work vs. socialization) [Wrong Planet.net, 2011].

In another forum an individual reflects on the effect of ADD on a past boyfriend who she notes was "hyper-focused" on her during the beginning of their relationship. Although there is not enough information on the post to identify whether or not this is the result of stimulants, we can see unfortunate negative effects of this hyper-focused state on the relationship [Wiki. answers. com].

Summary of the Side-Effects of Stimulants on Socialization

The effects of these prescription stimulant drugs are supposed to help reduce behaviours portrayed by many individuals with ADHD that seem off-putting in social situations such as impulsiveness, lack of focus, irritability, etc. Observers of individuals taking these prescription drugs may notice a more relaxed and concentrated individual after they have taken their prescription and they may assume that these characteristics are more normal and desirable for socialization. However, it is possible that a stimulant drugs' ability to increase concentration in individuals could also provide a negative effect on socialization as individuals with ADHD who take the drugs may find socialization a waste of their time and unimportant when compared to the task at hand. These individual may become overly focused and as a result may neglect social relationships and in turn decrease their sociability because of the effects of stimulant medication. If this side-effect goes unnoted and the individual continues to not feel like socializing while on the drug it can be detrimental to the individual's long-term social health.

In the younger population this side-effect could be particularly debilitating as it is at the younger ages that individuals learn to socialize appropriately and start to build a social base that can follow them throughout their life. In the adult population with ADHD withdrawing socially because of the use of stimulant drugs can negatively affect not only the adults with ADHD, but also their children, husband or wife, coworkers, extended family, etc.

Therefore, based on the evidence, it seems that there is indeed a severe risk to taking prescription medication for ADHD behaviours, at least in the way of social withdrawal. The question is then, if an individual finds these side-effects debilitating, and switching medication and reducing medication dosage isn't helping, should they stop using the drugs all together or would taking "drug holidays" outside of school/school work be enough down-time from the drug? It would seem that in some cases these methods may work for the individuals involved, however when it is possible to avoid drugs or reduce the amount taken for a problem, most professionals would likely recommend this method. This is likely why many recommend a combination of drugs and behavioural therapy to aid individuals in the way the drugs cannot, or to help them become less dependent on the drugs [Centers for Disease Control and Prevention, 2009; Conners, et al., 2001].

TOPIC #3: IS THIS REDUCTION IN SOCIALIZATION BENEFICIAL?

What Are the Benefits of a Reduction in Socialization?

We have established that in some cases individuals with ADHD may suffer the side-effect of social withdrawal when taking prescription stimulant medication. We have also established the negative consequences of social withdrawal on the individual and on those around them. However, the hyper-focus that often goes along with this reduced desire to socialize may provide some benefits to the individual. As noted above [Davis-Berman, and Pestello, 2010], some individuals on ADHD medications noted that in place of a desire to socialize was a desire to focus on school-work. Therefore, it is possible that this side-effect is not truly negative in all accounts, there could be a benefit to this side-effect when social withdrawal symptoms are paired with an increased focus (we can refer to this as "hyper-focused") on something positive (e.g. academic pursuits).

Indeed, authors Davis-Berman, and Pestello [2010] actually noted that although the social withdrawal documented by some individuals taking these prescription medications for ADHD could indeed prove to be a negative side-effect, the social withdrawal could also potentially be seen as a benefit for the individual. This benefit could come in the form of shifting focus away from social factors that would otherwise distract them from doing their work. The result would be an increased focus on their work and therefore an increase in their performance in work. In this respect the individual may be focused away from social activities, but at the same time, they do seem to be more focused on positive tasks like academic pursuits. Recall the individual who was quoted as saying "…when I was on medication for ADD, I didn't want to talk to my friends, I just wanted to do my homework" [Davis-Berman, and Pestello, 2010]. Also noted in the same study where we find this quote, was the reference to individuals taking "drug holidays" on the weekends and during breaks from school. The individuals who took these "drug holidays" realized that it seemed only necessary to use the medication to perform successfully in school [Davis-Berman, and Pestello, 2010].

Do Individuals with ADHD Taking Prescription Stimulant Medication Have an Advantage Over Others?

Davis-Berman, and Pestello [2010], also reported briefly on the trend of those without the diagnosis of ADHD trying to acquire stimulant medications in order to increase their ability to focus in school so that they could receive better marks. This trend is also noted by Advokat [2010]. Advokat [2010] briefly reflects on the abundant research performed on an increase in illicit use of ADHD medication by students in order to perform better in school by increasing their focus on studying and performing other otherwise mundane school tasks.

This increase in illicit use of ADHD medication of course does not provide proof that the medications will increase grades, but it does feed into the fact that individuals believe they are better at academic pursuits while on the medication even if they do not have ADHD. Whether this is true or is some sort of placebo effect is not within the scope of this particular study, but authors Davis-Berman and Pestello [2010], did note that of their participants with ADHD interviewed, all reported that their medication provided them with the ability to increase their concentration, focus and memory. They also noted that they earned better grades and overall performed better in school. Indeed, as mentioned in Whalen, and Henker's [1991] research, many researchers have noted that stimulants seem to facilitate academic functioning. So, do individuals with ADHD gain an advantage over others when they take these prescription medications?

The answer is "no", stimulant drugs do not provide individuals with ADHD with an advantage over others. Advokat [2010] notes that individuals with ADHD in college were recorded as having less self-control, were less organized and showed less discipline, procrastinated more and used significantly fewer coping strategies compared to their peers without ADHD. Other researchers' efforts to provide a clear analysis of the impact of stimulant medications on academic performance is also summarized in this research [Advokat, 2010]. According to their report, even with the use of stimulant medications, individuals diagnosed with ADHD do not constantly see an improvement in academic performance. To the contrary, according to these researchers, most individuals with ADHD fail classes and the majority does not enter college, or if they do, they are likely to drop out. Based on the measures used to typically assess academic achievements however, it is no wonder students with ADHD do not fare as well. Most testing situations require prolonged attention, work on mundane tasks and standardized learning which individuals with ADHD may have problems with. If we are to truly understand academic abilities in particular of individuals with ADHD we should be assessing them in a manner which is consistent to the way the individual learns and works. Perhaps we should take a leaf out of the research performed by Andrews, Bonta and Hoge on the "Risk, Need and Responsivity principles" [Andrews, Bonta, and Hoge, 1990]. If we were to use the Rick, Need and Responsivity principles we would determine the intensity of aid an individual may require (risk principle – e.g. match low cases with low intensity aid and high cases with high intensity aid), reduce the circumstances that negatively affect their behaviours and increase the circumstances that positively affect their behaviours (need principle) and match their learning style and abilities with the work to be done as opposed to using a standardized method (responsivity principle). If individuals with ADHD were able to learn and work in a way that was more conducive to their needs they may show higher levels of achievement than they would in situations that inhibit different methods of learning and working. Indeed, Advokat [2010] also reported that those with ADHD did not differ from those without ADHD in IQ scores and were able to meet the demands of college courses.

Perhaps those individuals diagnosed with ADHD who do accomplish higher rates of academic achievement do not show the same symptoms as others diagnosed with ADHD who do not achieve the same academic standards, perhaps they use different learning methods, perhaps using stimulants helps them concentrate and use learning methods that work for them but which others with ADHD have not mastered. Just as the population without ADHD are all individual learners and use individualized methods to achieve the goals and skills they desire, so too do individuals with ADHD. We are all individual and do not all learn the same way.

So What Benefits *Can* Stimulant Drugs Provide in Terms of Academic Achievement for Individuals With ADHD?

Stimulants may help those with ADHD access information they already had but were unable to access because of behavioural blocks such as inattention and inability to concentrate. It does not provide them with any miracle drugs that make individuals smarter or provide them with skills or knowledge they do not already have, it simply provides them with the ability to access the skills and knowledge they already have.

To shed more light on this topic we can turn to a study performed by Pelham et al. in 1990 [cited in Whalen, and Henker, 1991], where the researchers reviewed an individual with ADHD's ability to perform during baseball drills and games while taking methylphenidate. The researchers found that the participants did not show an increase in skill level (e.g. battering, throwing or catching) but they did note that there were "marked beneficial effects on attending and following the action" during the games. This research reveals that the medications did not provide the individuals with better baseball skills, but instead, provided them with better focus and attention to the game itself. In the same way, these drugs, when taken by individuals with ADHD, may help them perform better in their academic pursuits, but it is not because the drugs provide them extra skills that others do not have. Instead, the drugs provide them with a more level playing field by providing them with an ability most other individuals already have: the ability to focus on the task at hand.

So, Is It Just Those Who Have the Side-Effect of a Hyper-Focused State Who See an Increase in Performance?

With this all said, it seems as though individuals with ADHD who take prescription stimulant medication receive access to skills they cannot normally access on their own.

This may provide them with the ability to focus on studies and other achievements. However, as noted above, this does not always mean that individuals with ADHD who take stimulant drugs are able to attain higher levels in academics, sports or careers. What may provide individuals with ADHD an advantage is when the side-effects of social withdrawal are present and paired with the desire to hyper-focus on academics, sports or career. It is possible that this disregard for social ties may provide these individuals with an advantage over others who do not have ADHD and may be able to focus on tasks on their own but still be dedicated to social requirements such as spending time with family and friends. It may even prove to be an advantage over others with ADHD on stimulant medications who may be able to better focus, but still not feel the side-effects of social withdrawal and therefore, not disregard their social interactions in place of only focusing on work.

However, if this is true, we must ask ourselves, is the possibility of increased performance in school or other areas of performance such as sports or work worth the cost of reduced socialization? They are probably not. By neglecting social relationships individuals will likely lose close attachments like family, friends and may even diminish their ability to perform in the workplace or sports because they may not see the need to interact with others or they may not know how to appropriately interact with others if they have not socialized much in their earlier years. Social experiences and the desire to socialize are very important at younger ages as this is when individuals develop social skills.

These social skills are even more important for individuals with ADHD to grasp as studies have shown that individuals with ADHD have a hard time interacting appropriately in social situations and are often rejected by peers [Whalen, and Henker, 1991]. In a study performed by Whalen, and Henker [1991], the authors referred to a report by Cunningham et al. in 1985, where the researchers noted that children with ADHD spent less time observing their peers in social interaction circumstances, potentially diminishing their abilities (compared to others without ADHD) in interacting appropriately in social situations.

If we agree that social skills are too valuable to lose even in place of increased performance then those suffering from social withdrawal side-effects because of stimulant medications should consider alternative measures to deal with their ADHD symptoms. In such cases, perhaps an appropriate avenue to take would be to use behavioural therapy instead. The authors, Whalen, and Henker [1991] argue that medications administered to individuals with ADHD should actually rarely if ever be used. The authors make this argument because while they acknowledge that medication can be useful in reducing unwelcome behaviour often exhibited through symptoms of ADHD, they cannot help an individual with ADHD gain any new skills that they can apply to improve their lifestyle without drugs. Because of this, the authors argue that a better method would be to use behavioural therapy focused in particular on "building social repertoires and mastering self-regulation" [Whalen, and Henker, 1991].

It would seem that although medication is useful in reducing negative behaviours that may diminish an individual's chances at social interaction, which provides an increase in the individual's ability to socialize, some individuals suffer the side-effects of the medication and no longer feel like socializing. So, the chances of social inclusion may become more frequent through the use of the drug, but if the individual decides they do not wish to be in a social environment, then this conflicts with the possible social benefit provided by the drug. For this reason, drug treatment may be better used only in situations where focus on work or mundane tasks takes precedence. This way the individual is less likely to suffer from any reduced desire to socialize as they should not be socializing much in these situations. For situations where socialization is appropriate, it would be best if the individual was not taking the drugs, but in order to facilitate socialization, behavioural therapy may be used to aid the individual in acquiring appropriate social skills.

This strategy is most likely going to be useful for individuals dealing with ADHD earlier in life, later in life once individuals with ADHD have begun to understand their ADHD symptoms better, they may be able to train themselves to focus on tasks they deem as important and no longer require the assistance of medication or professional behavioural therapy except perhaps in extreme circumstances. For example, see this quote from an online forum posted by an individual with ADHD: "when it comes to tests such as the SAT or Midterms, I go into a hyper focus that I have trained myself to do" [Wiki.answers.com].

Therefore, this author believes that a combination of drug and behavioural therapy is best in most cases.

Conclusion

Throughout this chapter the goal has been to discuss, in terms of functionality, the benefits and the disadvantages of the most popular method used to help individuals deal with symptoms of ADHD: stimulant drugs.

Based on this discussion, it has become apparent that stimulant drugs can be a beneficial treatment method for those suffering the effects of ADHD symptoms, particularly inattention, hyperactivity and impulse control. It is believed that individuals with ADHD suffer from malfunction of brain chemicals which stimulate functions that provide impulse control, focus, attention, etc. These drugs work because they help regulate the functioning of these chemicals, allowing the individual to inhibit hyperactive and impulsive behaviour.

There are however, problems with this method of treatment, particularly there are side-effects that may occur with the use of these drugs. Although the type and severity of side-effects may vary depending on the individual, the drug and the dosage, it is possible that some side-effects may go unnoted and may be detrimental to an individual's well-being. In particular it was asserted that individuals suffering from the side-effect of social withdrawal may go unnoted because they are displaying symptoms that seem positive to onlookers; for instance, they may be focused on work or other positive tasks and be less disruptive to those around them. However, if an individual neglects social relationships because they are constantly focusing on other tasks, it may result in a detrimental effect to their relationships, their social abilities and other areas of their life where socialization is necessary (e.g. group work, team sports, family life, etc.).

Individuals taking these medications may be left in a hyper-focused state that disengages them from social activity. In small dosages this hyper-focused state may be beneficial to the individual as they are able to concentrate on tasks without the disruption of socialization. However, if over time, the individual continues in this state, we may see the negative results mentioned above. For this reason, it is important that if the individual does suffer from this side-effect that they either stop the drug treatment or take what are called "drug holidays", where they only take the drugs during times where focus is necessary and socialization is not.

In addition to the possible side-effect of reduced desire to socialize, individuals only using stimulant drugs for treatment of ADHD are simply masking the problems. Although these drugs may allow an individual to focus and maintain proper impulse control, they are not increasing skills in areas they may have difficulty in, such as socialization.

Individuals who have been diagnosed with ADHD have often shown difficulty in social situations. It is argued that individuals who display symptoms of ADHD often show less interest in observing their peers in social situations, and thus are less likely to understand social cues and appropriate socialization. So, even if the individual does not suffer from the side-effect of reduced desire to socialize, the drugs, although providing the individual with more appropriate behaviours for social interactions (e.g. more focus, less hyperactivity and more impulse control), do not provide them with any growth of social skills. It is for these reasons that this researcher, along with many other researchers and professionals in the field, recommend a multimodal treatment method for individuals suffering from symptoms of ADHD.

Multimodal treatment would provide the individual with the ability to use stimulant medication when necessary, but it would also provide them with behavioural therapy focused on proving them with skills they may find difficult to gain such as social skills, it is also useful to provide the individual with a better understanding of their symptoms and to find work and study methods that benefit them most. It is the hope that as the individual grows and continues to gain understanding and skills in these areas they may have struggled with, that their dependence on and use of stimulant medication may diminish.

As the research is scattered in the area of social withdrawal effects of stimulant medication on individuals with ADHD, it would be interesting for future research to focus on the effects of stimulant medication in particular on socialization throughout the lifespan of individuals diagnosed with ADHD. It would also be important to understand how a combination of stimulant treatment and behavioural therapy may differ in regards to social skills and abilities and overall satisfaction with life in comparison with individuals with ADHD simply taking stimulant medication. It would also be useful to see if either group was able to successfully diminish their use of stimulant medication later in life and what methods allowed them to do this.

Regardless of the results however, one thing is certain, there are many different treatments available for individuals trying to manage their ADHD symptoms and more treatments will likely be added to this collection and be modified as we learn more about this disorder. There is no one treatment that will work for all individuals however, and therefore each must undergo a trial and error process to find the treatment that works best for them. It is certain though, that there is much importance in the identification of side-effects of any treatment method. Each individual and those around them must take careful precautions to identify any side-effects and changes in behaviour, regardless of whether or not the change seems beneficial at the time. One true goal should always be the focus of any treatment: providing the individual with ADHD with a way to manage their symptoms in a manner that allows them to live a life without barriers.

REFERENCES

Advokat, C. (2010). What are the cognitive effects of stimulant medications? Emphasis on adults with attention-deficit/hyperactivity disorder (ADHD). *Neuroscience and biobehavioral reviews*, 34, 1256-1266.

American Psychiatric Association. (2012). American psychiatric association DSM-5 development: A 06 attention deficit/hyperactivity disorder. http://www.dsm5.org/ProposedRevisions/Pages/proposedrevision.aspx?rid=383#

Andrews, D. A., Bonta, J., and Hoge, R. D. (1990). Classification for effective rehabilitation: Rediscovering psychology. *Criminal justice and behavior*, 17(1), 19-52.

Breggin, P. R. (1998). Psycho-stimulant effects on children: A primer for school psychologists and counselors. AbleChild.org. http://ablechild.org/psycho-stimulant%20efect%20on%20children.htm

Breggin, P. R. (2001). Talking back to ritalin: What doctors aren't telling you about stimulants and ADHD (revised edition). Cambridge, MA: Da Capo Press.

Centers for Disease Control and Prevention. (2009). Social skills in adults with ADHD (WWK15). National Resource Center on ADIHD: A Program of CHADD. http://www.help4adhd.org/en/living/relandsoc/WWK15

Children and Adults with Attention-Deficit/Hyperactivity Disorder (CHADD). (2012). Understanding ADHD: How is ADHD treated? CHADD. http://www.chadd.org/AM/Template.cfm?Section=TreatmentandTemplate=/CM/HTMLDisplay.cfmandContentID=23669

Conners, C. K., et al. (2001). Multimodal treatment of ADHD in the MTA: An alternative outcome analysis. *Journal of the American academy of child and adolescent psychiatry,* 40(2), 159-167.

Davis-Berman, J. L., and Pestello, F. G. (2010). Medicating for ADD/ADHD: Personal and social issues. *International journal of mental health and addiction,* 8, 482-492.

Doggett, M. A., (2004). ADHD and drug therapy: Is it still a valid treatment? *Journal of child health care,* 8(1), 69-81.

Faraone, S.V., and Biederman, J. (2005). What is the prevalence of adult ADHD? Results of a population screen of 966 adults. *Journal of attention disorders*, 9, 384–391.

Feingold. (2008). History of ADHD as a recognized disorder. http://www.feingold.org/adhd-history.html

Hallowell, E. M., and Ratey, J. J. (1994). The evolution of a disorder. Excerpted from drive to distraction (Touchstone 1994). PBS frontline. http://www.pbs.org/wgbh/pages/frontline/shows/medicating/adhd/evolution.html

Hoffman, H. (2004). The Project Gutenberg EBook of Struwwelpeter: Merry takes and funny pictures. http://www.gutenberg.org/files/12116/12116-h/12116-h.htm

Kail, R. V., and Barnfield, A. (2009). Children and their development (first Canadian edition). Pearson Education Canada.

Low, K. (2010). How do stimulants for ADHD work? About.com. http://add.about.com/od/treatmentoptions/f/How-Do-Stimulants-Work.htm

Maxwell, A. (2011). Are some individuals diagnosed with ADHD prone to alcohol abuse? Consideration of two possible mediating factors for this susceptibility. *Journal of attention disorders*, XX(X), 1-4.

Moynihan, R., and Cassels, A. (2005). Selling sickness: How the world's biggest pharmaceutical companies are turning us all into patients. New York, NY: Nation Books.

Nauert, R. (2012). ADHD diagnoses up 66 percent since 2000. PsychCentral. http://psychcentral.com/news/2012/03/20/adhd-diagnoses-up-66-percent-since-2000/36229.html

Pearson, D. A., Santos, C. W., Roache, J. D., Casat, C. D., Loveland, K. A., Lachar, D., Lane, D. M., Faria, L. P., and Cleveland, L. A. (2003). Treatment effects of methylphenidate on behavioral adjustment in children with mental retardation and ADHD. *Journal of the American academy of child and adolescent psychiatry*, 42(2), 209-216.

Prediger, R. D. S., Pamplona, F. A., Fernandes, D., and Takahashi, R. N. (2005). Caffeine improves spatial learning deficits in an animal model of attention deficit hyperactivity disorder (ADHD) – the spontaneously hypertensive rat (SHR). *International journal of neuropsychopharmacology,* 8, 583-594.

Rapport, M. D., Stoner, G., DuPaul, G. J., Birmingham, B. K., and Tucker, S. (1985). Methylphenidate in hyperactive children: Differential effects of dose on academic, learning, and social behavior. *Journal of abnormal child psychology*, 13(2), 227-244.

Singh, I., (2008). ADHD, culture and education. *Early child development and care,* 178(4), 347-361.

Smith, B. H., Molina, B. S. G., and Pelham, W. E. Jr. (2002). The clinically meaningful link between alcohol use and attention deficit hyperactivity disorder. *Alcohol research and health*, 26, 122-129.

Smith, B. H., Pelham, W. G., Evans, S., Gnagy, E., Molina, B., Bukstein, O., Greiner, A., Myak, C., Presnell, M., and Willoughby M. (1998). Dosage effects of methylphenidate on the social behavior of adolescents diagnosed with attention-deficit hyperactivity disorder. *Experimental and clinical psychopharmacology,* 6(2), 187-204.

Spine Universe. (2010). Central nervous system (CNS) depressants and stimulants. http://www.spineuniverse.com/treatments/medication/central-nervous-system-cns-depressants-stimulants

Vanderschuren, L. J. M. J., Trezza, V., Griffioen-Roose, S., Schiepers, O. J. G., Van Leeuwen, N., De Vries, T. J., and Schoffelmeer, A. N. M. (2008). Methylphenidate disrupts social play behavior in adolescent rats. *Neuropsychopharmacology,* 33(12), 2946-2956.

Visser, S. N., Bitsko, R. H., Danielson, M. L., Perou, R., and Blumberg, S. J. (2010). Increasing prevalence of parent-reported attention-deficit/hyperactivity disorder among children --- United States, 2003 and 2007. Centers for disease control and prevention, 59(44), 1439-1443. http://www.cdc.gov/mmwr/preview/mmwrhtml/mm5944a3.htm?s_cid=mm5944a3_w

Weafer, J., Fillmore, M. T., and Milich, R. (2009). Increased sensitivity to the disinhibiting effects of alcohol in adults with ADHD. *Experimental and clinical psychopharmacology*. 17(2), 113-121.

Whalen, C. K., and Henker, B. (1991). Social impact of stimulant treatment for hyperactive children. Journal of learning disabilities, 24(4), 231-241.

Wiki.answers.com. *How does adult ADD-ADHD affect relationships with other adults and partners?* http://wiki.answers.com/Q/How_does_adult_ADD_ADHD_affect_relationships_with_other_adults_and_partners#ixzz216DIc3Jk

WrongPlanet.net. (2011). Retalin and social interaction. http://www.wrongplanet.net/postt180943.html

In: ADHD ISBN: 978-1-62417-107-9
Editors: R. Thompson and N. J. Miller

Chapter 2

FAMILY DYNAMICS, CONVERSATIONS AND ATTACHMENT PATTERNS: THE CONSTRUCTION OF ADHD

Rudi Dallos, Cordet Smart and Katie Denman
Programme Director and Professor of Clinical Psychology on the Doctorate in Clinical Psychology Training Programme at the University of Plymouth, Plymouth, Devon, UK

ABSTRACT

The paper offers a detailed case study of one family taken from a wider research programme investigating the role of family conversational and attachment processes in the development and maintenance of problems labelled as ADHD and self-harm. Individual narrative based attachment assessments and a semi – structured family interview were employed and included an exploration of the current and past problems, family identity, management of feelings, and a family sculpt. Analysis drew on conversational analysis (CA) to focus on the processes of meaning construction between family members. It also utilised the structured form of discourse analysis employed in the Adult Attachment Interview to help reveal defensive processes.

The findings suggested that individual attachment strategies both shaped and were in turn in maintained by the family conversational processes. Specific focus was on how the conversation processes could serve to manage significant attachment dilemmas, such as divided loyalties, triangulation and expressions of anger and protest in the child with the ADHD label.

INTRODUCTION

It might appear from referral rates in child mental health settings, and now increasingly in adult contexts, that there is a virtual epidemic of ADHD (NICE, 2006; Scharfstein, 2006). There are intense contemporary debates about whether and to what extent ADHD is a form of illness which has some biological or dispositional basis (Schore, 2003; Roy et al, 2004; NICE, 2006, Nylund, 2000). The clinical picture is quite complex and confusing in part because a similar presentation may be manifest in post-traumatic stress disorders, for example, resulting from children witnessing repeated conflicts and domestic violence (Schore, 1994 2003; Spatz – Wisdom, 1999; Vetere and Cooper, 2006). Because in clinical practice the diagnosis of ADHD often overlaps with conduct disorders, we will refer in this paper more broadly to problems of attention and conduct.

The problems described within the rubric of ADHD include hyperactivity, inability to concentrate, difficulties in regulating moods and not infrequently the concept has also been employed to include problems of anger (Vetere and Cooper, 2006, Scharfsein, 2006, Nylund, 2000). In diagnostic systems the process of classification involves lumping together behaviours that look similar and from there it is a small step to assume that these have a similar aetiology. However, a number of theoretical models question this assumption. For example, systems theory employs the concepts of equifinality in that what appear to be the same behaviours may in fact have been shaped by quite different be caused processes (Dallos and Draper, Weiner), . Further, difficulties may have been multiply determined by varying combinations of factors in different situations. In essence this helps us to differentiate between the surface aspects of behaviours and the underlying causal mechanisms.

A number of studies which indicate that young people diagnosed with ADHD and conduct disorders also display insecure attachment patterns (Fitz-Dotan, 2006; Clarke et al , 2002; Dow, 2006; Crittenden and Kulbotten, 2007). However, there are relatively few studies which appear to have focussed on the observation of parents' behaviour and in turn the parents own attachment patterns and histories which guide their parenting (Crittenden and Kulbotton, 2007P). Studies also suggest (Fitz- Dozen, 2006; Erdman, 1998; Kissgen et al, 2009; Mash and Johnson, 2005; Moretti et al, 1994) that parents demonstrate insecure attachments with indications that they display inconsistent responses to the child. There is evidence of an association of ADHD with children growing up in family environments where there is conflict and possibly violence between the parents and generally inconsistent parenting (Ladnier and Massanari, 2000, Dallos and Smart, 2011)). It is possible that ADHD, like many other severe problems, needs to be understood in terms of a complex interplay of the family dynamics and the parents' self –protective attachment strategies.

Both systemic and attachment perspectives are relevant to an understanding of ADHD but arguably both s have fallen short of their desired ambitions: Family therapy offers a picture of the complexity of family connections but falls short of showing how this relates to different kinds of inner worlds and problems. Similarly, attachment theory does not offer an understanding of the full complexity of the family processes that shape attachment patterns. It is being increasingly recognised that children, for example develop multiple attachment strategies for different attachment figures in their lives. Attachment theory has been regarded as taking a 'narrative turn' in its increasing emphasis on attempting to consider 'internal representations' of experience rather than the early emphasis on behaviour (Main et al, 1985). This emphasis on understanding and representing the world starts to connect attachment theory with social constructionist approaches which emphasise the centrality of meaning – making.

Social constructionist approaches to the exploration of problems emphasise that 'problems' do not have an objective existence but instead can be seen as creations in relational systems (Gergen,1999) Anderson et al (1986) refer to problem determined and problem saturated systems. A dilemma for research in clinical areas is how to refer to the phenomenon that we are interested in exploring. In the title to this paper we have used the label ADHD (Attention Deficit Hyperactive Disorder). Unfortunately the use of this diagnostic category leads us into making some assumptions about the nature of this condition, including what causes it and how it may be maintained. These assumptions are largely that it has an organic origin, possibly related to some hereditary, genetic factors and that these may be triggered or aggravated by social contexts , such as stress, high level of inter-personal conflict and arousal (Nylund, 2000, NICE 2006).

All of these assumptions are questionable and have been questioned (Clarke et al 2002, Erdman, 1998, Mash and Johnson, 2005). However, they appear to inform the dominant understandings of both professionals and family members.

AIMS OF THE STUDY

The broad aim of the study was to explore the contribution that a conversational analysis of family dynamics offers to an understanding of the development and maintenance of attachment patterns in the members of a family. Broadly this follows Bolwby's ( ) proposition that secure attachment develop in family contexts characterised by 'open' as opposed to 'closed' patterns of communication.

The varieties of qualitative analysis which are available for research have been develop predominantly to explore the accounts and experiences of individuals.

An exception is Conversational Analysis which combines the emphasis from Discourse analysis on 'rhetorical' strategies, for example, how family members attempts to influence and persuade each other (Gale, 2010, Hepburn and Wiggins, 2007, Sutherland and Strong, 2011) offers a numbers of key interpretative frameworks for analysing conversations. Conversational Analysis can be seen to share features with the analysis the pragmatics of communication which inspired early family therapy (Watzlawick et al).

The specific aims of the study were to explore the nature of the conversations in a family where ADHD is a presenting problems. The intention of the analysis was to consider how:

1. The conversational process could be seen to be shaped or influenced by the attachment strategies identified for each family member.
2. To consider how in turn the nature of the conversation served in turn to shape and maintain the attachment patterns of the family members.
3. To indicate points of potential change for the family conversational dynamics and attachment patterns for the family members.

METHOD

A single case study design was employed with one family where the young person in the family had a diagnosis of ADHD. The findings reported feature an analysis of a semi – structured interview conducted with the family and are supported by Adult Attachment and semi- structured interviews with each member of the family.

1. Family interview - this was intended both to elicit information about the meanings held by family members and also to elicit their characteristic patterns of conversational interaction. The interview included the following: a discussion of how they regarded themselves as a family – similarities and differences to other families, their explanations of the problems, family patterns managing feelings, including how comfort is offered when family are ill of emotionally distressed, trans- generation al patterns in relating and how emotions are managed, corrective and explicative scripts in terms of how the parents have incorporated or attempted to change elements of their own child experiences and how this shaped their attitudes to parenting. The interview ended with a reflective discussion of how their experiences together had shaped them as individuals, as a family and the implications of this for their future lives as individuals and as a family.

A family genogram and a family sculpt with coins was also employed to elicit further information about their perceptions and beliefs regarding changes in their relationships over time, a time line of significant events that had occurred in the family. All of the interviews were video taped and transcribed verbatim. The transcription utilised key features of the notation employed in Conversational Analysis (Gale, 2010),

2. The Adult Attachment Interview with the Diane and the step-father (Peter) and the Transition to Adulthood Attachment Interview (Crittenden, 2009) with the two teenage children.
3. Semi – structured interviews which explored the details of the particular problems being experienced by family members and also an open – ended interview to explore aspects of their individual and shared experiences.

These two individual interviews were employed to provide an indication of the attachment strategies (styles) of each of the family members and also to indicate their personal understanding, especially of the problems.

ANALYSIS

The analysis progresses in a series of over-lapping stages:

1. The dominant discourse themes under-pinning the family's understandings of their problems, especially in relation to ADHD.
2. The relational processes in terms of how the family members engaged in conversation and interacted to produce their shared discourses. Broadly this focused on the processes of meaning construction in the family and employed a CA framework to explore the patterns of conversation, such as amount of talking, interrupting, claiming the floor and also how meanings were constructed and contested. Specifically this featured: epistemic claims – who claimed to be right, supporting and contesting meanings, discursive strategies, such as connoting self as a victim, invoking illness models, claiming the moral high - ground.
3. The relational and emotional dynamics which appeared to under-pin the family conversational and relational processes, for example how meanings were contested, differences expanded and resolved. This analysis attempted to integrate features of the structured discourse analysis employed in the AAI. This is a 'top-down' form of discourse analysis which employs a repertoire of constructs derived from attachment theory to indicate the types of defensive processes which people are seen to be utilizing in order to manage their attachment needs.

FAMILY IN THE STUDY

The family contained a young person who had a formal diagnosis of ADHD and had been in contact with the NHS (National Health Service) Child and Adolescent Mental Health Services (CAMHS). The young person (Rick) was 16 years of age, and his brother (Keith) was 14. We were also able to interview their Diane, Diana, and step-father, Peter. The family were referred to us through a local CAHMs team, and were sent a letter asking whether they would like to participate. Key information and names have been changed in line with ethical requirements.

Rick was described by the parents and himself as having had considerable problems at school and also at home in terms of disruptive and angry behaviour. He was excluded from a number of schools and eventually Diane sought assistance from her GP and social services who were said to have been rather unhelpful. Diane had experienced a volatile and at times violent relationship with their father Anthony and when she left him, when Rick was aged 3. He moved away to live abroad for two years but returned continued to have contact and was described by Diane and Peter to have subsequently caused them considerable problems with at times violent altercations.

ATTACHMENT STRATEGIES

Rick: Oredominantly demonstrated a dismissive strategy (A: 4 – 6 - compliant /self-reliant) though occasionally showed some pre-occupied patterns when he became agitated, confused and angry when discussing his natural parents' relationship. He also showed disorientation, and unresolved dismissed traumas regarding his own self – harm and his parents' divorce.This were indicated by repeated statements that he was not surer if his memories were real, what he really thought or whether he could belileve what people had said to him.

Diane: Showed a mixed pattern of both employing dismissive as well as pre-occupying attachment strategies (A4/C2 - Dismissive Compliant and Pre-occupied Disarming). She also displayed several unresolved traumatic states: One of these appeared to be a dismissed trauma regarding Terry's domestic violence and threats and also his self harm in front of the family. This possibly also contained some displaced trauma in that she was extremely concerned about the influence it had on the children. In addition she seemed to hold a pre-occupying trauma regarding Ricks self harm, where he cut himself with a knife. The traumatic memories had an efect of breaking into her account at tines so that she would become aroused, agitated, used strong and evocative language and images.

Peter: Peter's AAI indicated an overall dismissive strategy (A 4/6 - Compliant and self – reliant).

Keith: His TAAI appeared to display an unresolved, dismissed trauma regarding his father's self harm. Overall he also displayed a Dismissive Attachment Pattern (A 2/4 - Socially facile – compliant).

Analysis of Family Interview

Discourse Themes:

Four discourse themes appeared throughout the family interviews:

- Are we normal: Definitions of 'normal' Family Life.
- Medical and biology discourse - personality and problems as due to heredity.
- Responsibility and free – will.
- Family problems and conflicts.

Though distinc these themes were also inter-dependent and the conversation would seguay from one to another as explanations of the problems and justifications of their actions and positions were ofered. Of particular interest to our analysis were 'contested moments' where, for example the implications of one of the themes escalated and was countered by the entrance of another theme. These episodes of contestation also appeared to be related to the emotional and attachment dynamics in the family such that strategies for resolving tension, blame and guilt became evident at these moments. In particular the major axis around which these contested meanings seemed to rotate was between discourses of biological and heredity based explanations and those of free – will and social factors, such as family conflicts and distress.

The themes are presented in the order in which they emerged during the family interview. This is both to capture the directions of the narrative of the family conversation but also to indicate how their conversation progressed through a general description of themselves as a family to specific explanations of the problems and what they saw as leading them to be not 'normal' in some ways.

Are We Normal : Definitions of 'Normal' Family Life

This discourse theme consisted of a thread of conversations regarding whether they were a 'normal' as opposed to atypical family. The key propagator of the view that they were not 'normal' was initially Keith and this was defended against by Diane and Rick. A sub-text of this discussion was that their lack of normality was due to Rick's difficult behaviour. Though Rick's responsibility for their problems was not specifically stated, nevertheless as the conversation progresses it seemed that Rick had an important investment in the family being seen as normal since if it was not then he was to blame.

RD: Just to sort of start off I mean how would you sort of describe yourselves as a family…what kind of things do you like doing together/ how would you describe yourself as different to other families you know….

Diane: (.4) {Peter turns to look at Diane, Diane then turning first to Rick and then Keith and laughter} (.5) Who do you want to answer this?

RD: Anybody that's just an open question

Diane : Would you like to answer that question {to Rick}? =

Keith : Well we don't really do much as a whole family, different opinions

RD: You don't now or you used to but?

Keith: We never really did much as a whole family:

Diane: .HHH HEHEHEHAHAHA {loud, shrill laughter})

Keith: What

Diane: HEHEHEHEH

Keith: What

Diane oh: Bless ahe

RD: Is that different to other families you know or similar do you know some families that do loads of things together

Keith: No not really no {Diane looking intently at Keith}

RD: No

Keith: {spoken softly} But we don't in all fairness if we normally go out its normally me mum and dad {turning to Diana}

Diane: Oh yea but that's only now that's only the last year really ^

Keith: No its inaudible) ( ) not no its not

In this very first passage Peter looks to Diane to initiate the responding. She then invites Rick in to speak, looking at him and Keith in turn. He declines and his brother steps in to suggest that they are unusual in that they do not do very much together. Diane then engages in a contesting of this definition of the family by making counter-claims that they do things together and then engages in several bouts of very loud, shrill almost demonic laughter. The intensity of this laughter suggests that the mild accusation that they are not 'normal' from Keith may have triggered some anxiety about the family and possibility her own responsibility as a mother. One effect of his mother's intense response appears to be that keith softens his response by stating, softly ' in all fairness' . Diane appears to develop this minimising further by her emphasis on we don't 'now' to sussgest that this is a recent state and later suggests that it is due to a normal developmental family stage of adolescents claiming more independence. This initial passage appears to represent both a core concern and dynamics in the family in that it appears to underlie a concern about whether they are 'normal' and the sub-text that one of the core causes of this abnormality is due to Rick's behaviour. It also indicates that the Diane takes, and is allowed to take, the lead throughout the interview in responding to the questions first, saying most and also prompting responses from the other family members. Diane repeatedly invites the children to comment she also appears to be very concerned to act as an arbitrator of what meaning about family life is conveyed.

Very early in the family interaction a second process appears and then can be seen repeatedly which involves the children and especially Rick turning to her for information and confirmation. In particular Rick appears to be unsure of his own thinking and Diane assists him to think along with him inviting her to assist him:

RD: I mean my other question is a broader one about how you see yourselves as similar or different to other families, ...

Diane: Ummhhmh (4), uhmh

Peter: Personally I can't do that because (.) erm I know of no other family directly that has teenage boys so I've no bench mark and I came from came from a small and disjointed family anyway so I kind of came into fatherhood not really knowing very much about parenting and families anyway {looking over to Diane} and there's no there's no family that we're close to that have children of the same age =

Rick: Joan and Harry =

Peter : We don't spend any time with Joane and Harry

Rick: Mum goes there (inaudible)

Diane: Yeah ^ I think we're probably I think it's probably on a par I think there are families that do more things together where the children are for some you know =

Rick : We are *not* ^ {looking at Diane} like a dysfunctional family (Diane: mm) we are not really like in any we don' t kind of no one =

Diane: We're not dysfunctional or we are?[

Rick: No ( ) [Diana *No*_^, I don't think we are =

Rick: { looking at Diane} No we're not we're not some families, sometimes I imagine don't really have much contact with at all I suppose we <u>do</u> em but (.6)

Diane: {looking at Int.} We always eat dinner together every night =

Rick: Yea....

RD: Is that different to other families you know or similar do you know some families that do loads of things together

Keith : No not really no

Diane: We don't do very much as a four now but that's mainly because Rick is exercising his right as a teenager to follow his own path and that's fine em I think I Peter and I understand that Keith is coming to terms with it because he's not quite a tee.. you know he is a teenager but he's not old enough to kind of always have his own independence at 14 so for example the four of us are going out tonight but Rick has decided he doesn't want to come so he's not coming......

In this sequence it is possible to see that Peter starts by offering a side-stepping of the question of normality by saying that he has no bench-mark regarding other families and further develops this by saying that his own family was 'disjointed' so he cannot hold a clear perspective or legitimate opinion. In effect this is a sort of auto- disqualification of having an opinion which also serves to enable him to avoid giving an opinion or stating his position.

In the next passage we see that this strategy may be related to his anger at Rick's behaviour and also his wanting to support Diane. Furthermore, Diane seeks further support for this view by referring to this being an understanding that she and Peter hold. Diane also shows here how she uses a strategy of 'speaking for other people' in that she makes this allusion to knowing how Peter thinks and also forcefully explaining Rick's mind in that he is 'exercising his right'. This looks like a common feature of many families in that the Diane is not only the family spokes – person but also the family psychologist in being the one who knows what people think and feel and hence can interpret and explain their actions.

A further sequence illustrates how the question of Rick gaining independence and his own wish to portray the family as 'normal is developed:

Diane: {to Rick} you would ^ *I think if you had your choice* you would have your dinner in your bedroom if you could (1.2)

Rick: (inaudible, rubbing chin) Well it's good to have it with somebody

Diane: {looking at Rick throughout the next sequence} I know it's good {Laugh} *intellectually* you know it's good but

Rick: Be more convenient =

Diane: It would be more convenient .{laughter}...You'd probably eat more if I let you[

Peter : *but you NEVER WANT TO DO IT*

Diane : Yea you never {Laughter} so

Peter: You come down as late as possible gobble {Diane laughter} > it and then BUGGER OFF AS QUICKLY AS POSSIBLE

Diane: a he he he he he {Diane smiling and looking at both her sons in turn}

Peter : turn around and say , yeah you can sit there and say it's a really good thing that we have dinner together as a family BUT YOU'RE LYING ^ THROUGH YOUR TEETH CAUSE ACTUALLY

Diane: he he he he he

Rick : {quietly} Yeah I know it's a good thing

Peter: But you object

Rick: I object but I

RD: In principle in principle

Peter: ok that's honest that's honest {raised palms – accepting}

In this passage Rick appears to continue to support the proposition that the family is normal and that in fact he does not simply want to be out of it and that he does like to have his dinner with other family members. At first this is contested by Diane as a 'theoretical stance and then very forcefully by Peter as Rick 'lying through his teeth'. This is a starkly angrier tone that the usually rational position taken by Peter and possibly contains with it some of the anger regarding Rick's previous 'misdemeanours'. Diane appears to attempt to soften this angry statement from Peter by casting it as a humorous passage by laughing. Rick then eventually responds or capitulates, by agreeing that he 'in principle' he supports being together and this agreement or capitulation by Rick to accept their definition is then accepted by Peter leading to a closure as being 'honest'. This being in contrast to the earlier accusation of Rick that he was lying through is teeth. There appears to be a joint placatory movement at this in that RD also becomes drawn in by stressing 'in principle and then Peter responds by a mild capitulation that what Rick is now saying is honest.

Medical and Biology Discourse - Personality and Problems as Due to Heredity

Related to the discourse regarding 'normality' was the conceptualisation of the problems in the family as related to underlying biological causation and inherited personality. This was broadly related to the medical definitions of ADHD or borderline personality disorder. In particular this discourse centred on the similarities between Rick and his biological father Anthony. This discourse also contained ideas of personality and inherited personality characteristics. Importantly woven through the family conversation in which these ideas were expressed there was a thread of a contested discourse that self – control and choice could over-ride the biological explanations. However, the contest between these two discourses was not resolved and a lack of resolution, a sort of not – knowing and lingering uncertainty. This was at times connected to a sense of exasperation and of feeling let down by professional services for not being able to provide clear answers for them.

> Diane: I often say when he's sometimes been a bit despairing I often say you're half mine so you've got other things as well you know you haven't I don't mean that I'm got all the good and that his dad's all the bad I don't mean that but sometimes, sometimes I think Rick has been concerned that things have happened to his dad will happen to him and the things that have not gone right for his dad will not go right for him because you know he thinks it's set in stone that all of that stuff will automatically be his fate as well I mean...
>
> *RD: I mean do you all agree on this that that Rick takes after his dad?*
>
> *Rick* : Unanimous YES {looking at Diane} so we can just
>
> Keith: hhh
>
> Diane: {looking at Rick and then RD} He's physically like him he's definitely emotionally like him and there are some very strong genes that run in that family that Rick has definitely inherited so you know......(3).
>
> *RD: Physical similarities often set off you know chains of thoughts don't they if a baby looks like one parent you know sometimes a story develops*
>
> Diane: Yeah, well actually the physical resemblance <u>isn't</u> that strong {looking at Rick}

Rick: [There's the eyes there =

Diane: You've got the same colour eyes

Rick : Well eyes, its not just the colour of eyes though its not just the colour of eyes though, is it ? =

Diane: yeah

Rick : It's not just the *colour* of someone's eyes that makes them follow in someone's footsteps = {looking at Diane , smiling}

Diane: No

Rick: It's the *DESPAIR* ^ in them.. , laughter }

Diane: You don't < say that ...{laughter}

In this passage it is possible to see the shared family construction that Rick has inherited traits from his father and that this is fully accepted by Rick. Again in this passage we can see Diane speaking and interpreting Rick's mind. Importantly she is suggesting that Rick feels he is trapped in a fatalistic view that history will repeat itself and that he will turn out to be like his father. This is followed by discussion about inheritance and appearance and that Rick is not physically so like his father.

This passage comes to a climax with a poignant remark by Rick that it's the despair in his father's eyes that leads him to follow him! This also appears to underlie his connection with, and caring for his father.

Diane's next remark that 'you don't say that' appears to a response to Rick saying something that he doesn't usually say, or perhaps something new as a result of this interview? Omissions in conversations can be as important as explicit content and here, as elsewhere in the family interview, the issue of the attachment dilemma faced by Rick in being close to his father in the context of the antagonism towards his father from his other and step-father is never pursued.

At the point above as Rick talks about responding to his father's despair, Diane appears to respond by emitting an enigmatic response – 'you don't say that'. Is she trying to say Rick 'must' not say this, 'should not' or that she is saying that he has not said this before?

Either way it does not invite further exploration of his poignant remark from Rick. Perhaps taking their cue from the Diane the other embers of the family likewise do not pursue this.

RESPONSIBILITY AND FREE – WILL

Following a few further exchanges about genes and hair colour Peter starts to contest the idea of hereditary factors with a discourse about responsibility for actions and free – will:

> Peter: ... {rest of family quiet no attempt to interrupt}Yes, Rick shares *a lot* of personality traits with er with Anthony but does also have ehm other stuff which comes from Diana and you know so it's not, it's not fair to say, it's *too easy* to say that it's you know he's a clone and therefore you know it's all pre-ordained and that sort of thing its very much erm. I do believe in ehm free will and you know making conscious decisions and changing cycles of behaviour and so on and so forth { gesticulating with hands dfor emphasis} and there's a degree of awareness em that that Rick has that Anthony *certainly doesn't have* and never had, hhh em in Anthony's family the, the resolution for the problem was that Anthony left home and went to live with his grandparents because he couldn't, he couldn't live with his with his own parents em and that kind of you know to be *fair at the time* they, they didn't know what they were *doing* and and em.. (5).

In this passage Peter engages in a number of different strategies. He contests the argument that Rick's behaviour is largely due to genes inherited from Anthony by first noting that inheritance comes from two parents, so Rick is also like his wife Diane. Secondly, he contests it by referring to free – will and conscious choice in changing behaviour. He points out by making a claim to know that Rick has more insight than his father, which is both a complement but also a further demand for Rick to take more responsibility for his behaviour. Furthermore, Peter here also makes a claim to know about Diana's ex-partner.

This theme of inheritance and free will is continued further by Diane:

> Diane: There weren't the child services then, Anthony was *trawled* before psychiatrists and psychologists for the whole of his childhood and when he got to about nine *his mother took to her ^ bed* she was on severe tranquilizers. When Anthony got to about nine she threw her hands in the air

and said actually I can't understand this child I can't deal with it you know he was violent and he was quite aggressive and *quite ^ a difficult child to raise* {laughter}in a time when they didn't *know*. I think Anthony probably had ADHD as well, a mild personality disorder and I think that they didn't actually know how to cope with it. So he was packed off to live with an *INCREDIBLY*_indulgent aunt who didn't do him any favours at all and arguably it set a course really for the rest of his life and he's never really found life terribly easy, has he? {turning to look at Rick} he's still on his own and you know he's had a succession of relationships that for one reason or another have never worked out for him =

Peter: ye yea but that's something that I've also seen because my brother had quite a lot of problems and when he was young my parents did you know a huge amount of hand wringing and they trawled *HIM* before all kinds of educational psychologists and you know various things > non of whom had the faintest idea, the closest they could get was borderline personality disorder which does not really ^ help.... basically we don't know but he's not quite right {smiling, laughter also Diane joins}

Peter and Diane in this sequence appear to develop each other's discourses about the relevance of inheritance and biological traits and relate this to aspects of troubled experiences in both of their families Significantly, both of them mention borderline personality disorder as an explanation though it is unclear whether this helped.

However, there is also introduced alongside this a theme that the biological traits may also be influenced by social processes, for example that the auntie's 'incredible indulgence', did not do Anthony ' any favours'. Likewise, Peter refers to his parents doing a lot o 'hand wringing' which appears dismissive of the value of concern and as indicated elsewhere in this family interview (and the individual interviews) that taking a form, no nonsense stance is seen as necessary in such cases, and by extension with Rick.

There appears to be a continuing processes whereby discourses of biology and inheritance are continually contested by the theme of responsibility and that personality traits cannot simply explain behaviour and , especially problems of both of the children's temper. This can be seen further in the discussion of temper and anger as a 'red mist'. In this sequence it is also possible to see how Rick supports a conversation which locates problems and anger in his brother, possibly since this eases the weight of the blame all falling on him.

Diane also distances herself very forcefully from such temper being anything like her temperament. Indirectly this again suggests that this probably is inherited for their father, Anthony.

LACK OF CONTROL OF TEMPER – RED MIST

Peter: Keith also has a lot of personality traits that he shares with his mother but he also has a lot in common with Freddy {their terrier dog....}

Diane: (to Rick) Keith does have Anthony's

Rick: [Stubborn attitude and temper] =

Keith: [get frustrated]

Diane: you *do* have a *FOUL TEMPER* and it's got you into an *AWFUL LOT OF TROUBLE* and I really *don't* have a foul temper

Rick: disregard for authority=

Diane: and I'm not stubborn

Peter: No that's true... No actually Anthony is, is *far more fearful* of authority (4).

Rick: Is he?

Peter: Yeah

Keith: What do you mean by that?

Peter: Well Anthony will fall into line very quickly if he thinks that there is an unstoppable force that's going to land on him, whether it's the tax man

Diana: a bit like yea a bit like you {to Rick}

Peter: ... or the police Anthony falls into line very quickly when it comes to authority, Rick absolutely doesn't

Diane: really doesn't,] the red mist comes down with Rick and actually it's like being hit with a hammer because you know he doesn't think em =

Keith : shut up now

Diane: you don't think consequences, consequences because actually once the red mist has come down you don't care what happens to you {looking at Keith} and em you know it quickly escalate
Peter: Keith 's very sorry about 48 hours later

Diane: laugh

Peter: and by that time its too late

Diane: The shit has hit the fan. {looking at Keith} .....

Keith: I did apologise to you after=

Diane: After, *AFTER* you have been an idiot (6) that's definitely a characteristic they share with their dad.

PROBLEMS RELATED TO FAMILY RELATIONAL ISSUES AND CONFLICTS

This theme captured notions of possible links between Rick's problematic behaviours and conflicts and distress in the family. In particular Diane mentions that Rick was aged three when the worst conflicts and distress between her and his father Anthony was taking place. However, this discourse was not developed despite prompts from RD in the interview. Instead, sources of conflict were connected to Rick's school situations and a recourse to ideas that there was something fundamentally unusual about Rick (biological and heredity discourse).

RD: right so at that time of that first exclusion it was just the three of you at that time and you'd separated from Anthony about a year ago ?

M: Yeah. But the problems with the playschool were while I was still married to his dad while I was still with him ..... Well ^ I mean it's quite a em melodramatic em statement to say that we were excluded they, they said that (.3)

Peter : Don't come back is {laughter}

Diane: yeah well they did they did say =

Rick : Exclusion is temporary , I wasn't outcast at three (M: mm) I wasn't outcast at three I think they probably just said something along the lines of...

Keith: Your EXPELLED {laughter , looking straight and directly said to Rick}

Diane: Yeah please don't please don't bring him ^ back (laugh)

Peter: > WE WOULD YEAH WE WOULD PREFER YOU TO TAKE YOUR SON SOMEWHERE ELSE............. {laughter} ....

This sequence starts with Diane making a reference to still being with the boy's father at the start of Rick's problems at school. However, this is immediately following by the nature of the exclusion itself. A process that recurred can be seen then in which a form of 'black humour' develops in jokes initiated by Peter about how Rick was asked 'not to come back' . There is laughter regarding this and Diane and Keith join in. The laughter here seems to serve a very interesting process in that it possibly conveys some anger and irritation fro Peter but in a manner which is disguised. His manner of conveying this is that the value of is talk, speed and emphasis heightens as he talks in contrast to a relatively flat tome he uses at other times. Interestingly, though Diane joins in the laughter her next response is to emphasise positive features of Rick, such as how beautiful he was as a baby:

Diane: Rick, Rick was em the most beautiful little boy absolutely gorgeous *but* Rick ...would *obsess* about things so he had *complete obsessions* about certain things and when it was trains he would obsess about *trains* he wouldn't talk about anything but *trains* he wouldn't watch a programme about anything except *trains* > I read him a good night story[Keith . Thomas the Tank engine] every night but it had to be about *trains* and he > wouldn't go in the car because he wanted to go in the *train* and then if we did go in the train we had to go somewhere where there was a *train line* near so that he could see some *trains* and *this is how* and then when the *train* phase stopped it became *dinosaurs*

Peter: I joined on dinosaurs.. {the family laughs}..............................

Rick: This might be a silly questions?, When I was obsessing about trains, what did I say ? I never had any intelligence of them ^ , what could I say about them ^? , was I running about manically shouting train ^?

Diane: What happened was =

Rick What could I say about them ?

Diane: {laught} cos you were obsessing, when they had the train set, which they always do, the train set because your domain................

The sequences ends with what appears to be a re-invoking of a biological discourse and frames the problem as within Rick.

Starting for discussing his beauty Diane then moves into a contrasting discourse of some fundamental temperamental flaws , which suggest that he has some form of obsession compulsive disorder.

Following this discussion RD attempts to probe again for evidence of alternative relational discourses:

RD: Can I just ask you I mean what was going on through that period I mean what were the stresses .. in what ways did you and the boys try and sort of find a bit of comfort …?

Diana: em what happened was that I, I did come to the conclusion actually, that my, my marriage was over and I needed to leave and I can't pretend that nothing was going on that they (the children) would have picked up on, especially Rick, a lot went on and I needed to leave. A lot went on that they should neither have seen or heard. By this time their dad was beginning to become quite unhinged > f he was here he would say that he was doing a job that he hated, he really couldn't cope with family life and by this time I think he hated me em. (3). He didn't after I left but he did before he left if you know what I mean {laugh}………….. he became increasingly ^ agitated and quite aggressive and I there was only about 6 months of that when Keith was very young and then I reached that point where I knew for my safety and for theirs I had to go ………..And that was that was hard because I just took the kids he wouldn't have left the house so they were taken out of their house we lived with a friend for 3 weeks and then I found my own home. Now all through that time > I was quite together, I mean I fell apart after the separation but I, I tried to keep it together as a mum and my parents were quite supportive and I had a best friend who was very supportive and she had two children and so we lived with her for a bit =

Keith: Who are you talking about Sue ?

Diana: Sue… .hh so it was it wasn't all death and destruction but it was a *very* unsettling time and then I was on my own for < about 8 or 9 months and then I met Peter so..

Diane: Do you want me to help you?

Diane described the split up with the children's father Anthony as a very difficult period and suggested that there was violence and ' events' which the children should not have seen or heard. This is followed by her describing how Anthony was appearing to have become 'unhinged'. Diane appeared to be on the point of making some causal connections between these events and Rick's state of mind at the time and his subsequent problems. There is a twin emphasis on this period having been hard but followed immediately by an emphasis on how she managed to cope with the help of a good friend.

RD makes a further attempt to invoke a discussions of psychological and relational factors that might be employed to explain Rick's difficulties:

RD: I'm not trying to lead your conversation …but children do often do collecting as a way of sort of comforting themselves …..in times of stress ….as a way of distracting themselves from things that are not very nice …… how did things develop did anyone else have problems did they go away for a while did they come back?

Diana: No I think the problem was definitely for Rick the problem was definitely school. and I think Rick's whole school life up until really very recently was a very unhappy experience and a very negative experience

RD: Do you Do you agree with your mum?

Rick: Yea definitely

RD: What was what made it unhappy for you?

Rick: er loneliness and insecurity in

Keith: Bullies...

RD: (to Rick) Looking back on it now do you have ideas=

Rick: Yeah many.

RD; Can you say ?

Rick: (0.6) er well I suppose when I was young em I can see myself doing that like well I suppose the things that people do wrong change during the kind of their own show something that you've done wrong in a social group a while ago would be (0.4) er there are certain things that I would ^ see myself doing and imagine as being wrong but I can't really put my finger on why they're wrong or why they're not socially acceptable

RD: Do you mean the other kids thought you were a bit unusual? What do you think was the main thing that made you seem unusual, in their eyes?

Rick: I suppose it's just a bit too old really, I can't put my finger on it.. =

RD: Too much of a swat, collecting things?

Diane: Do you want me to help you?=
Rick: I was never like ^ attention seeking ? {looking to mum} (.5)

Diane: < Yeah. You would attention seek but not in any traditional way. You ^ would just do things that were (4). The only word I can use that they use nowadays is kind of random.

Table 1. Transcript Notation

Symbol	Indicates
(.8)	pauses in tenths of seconds
CAPITAL	Words in capitals are uttered louder than surrounding talk
{ looks to}	Actions, such as turning to others, eye contact etc)
[ ]	Start or ending of overlaps in talk
> <	Shifts in speed of talk, faster or slower
Hhhhh	significant breathing out, or in if preceded by a
Becau -	Hyphen indicates a sudden cut – off or self interpretation of the sound
Dr ^ ink	A ^ indicates a marked rise in pitch
=	Latched relationship between two utterances, no silence at all between them
Underline	Indicates stress or emphasis
( )	Talk to obscure to transcribe

From Gale (2010).

In this last sequence Diane directs the conversation to problems at school and again with a statement of his unhappiness at school. This is related to the earlier discussion that Rick's obsessive behaviours caused these problems at school. However, when Rick is asked about his own ideas to explain these events he appears to become disorientated and confused about what exactly he might have been doing wrong. At this point, as happened frequently in the interview Diane intervened to offer to help him out and to explain his actions for him. However, what is offered is a somewhat enigmatic explanation of his actions being ‘random’, which potentially puts them beyond explanation or being accountable.

REFERENCES

Ainsworth,M.D.S. (1989) Attachments beyond infancy. *American Psychologist*, 44: 709-716.

Anderson, H., Goolishan, H.A. and Windermand, L.(1986) Problem determined systems: toward transformation in family therapy, *Journal of Strategic and Family Therapy,* 5*(4) :* 1-13.

Anolli, L. and Balconi, M. (2002) Adult attachment interview, thematic analysis, and communicative style in families with substance disorder. *Psychological Reports,* 90:279-299.

Bowlby, J. (1973) Attachment and Loss, vol.1 Separation , New York: Basic Books.

Bowlby, J. (1988) A secure base: clinical applications of attachment theory. New York: Basic Books London:Tavistock.

Byng - Hall, J. (1995) Rewriting Family Scripts. London: Guilford Press.

Clarke, L. , Ungerer, J., Chahoud, K., Johnson, S. And Stiefel, I. (2002) Attention deficit hyperactive disorder is associated with attachment insecurity. *Clinical Child Psychology and Psychiatry,* 7(2) : 179 – 198

Crittenden, P.M. (2009) Family Relations Institute, 9481, SW 147 St., Miami, FL 33176.

Crittenden, P. M. (2006). A dynamic-maturational model of attachment. *Australian and New Zealand Journal of Family Therapy, 27,* 105-115.

Crittenden, P.M. and Kulbotten, G.R. (2007) Familial contributions to ADHD: An attachment perspective. *Tidsskrift for Norsk Psykologforening. 44*:1220 – 1229.

Crittenden, P. and Dallos, R. (2009) All in the family: Integrating Attachment and Family Systems Theories. *Clinical Child Psychology and Psychiatry,* 14(3): 389-409.

Dallos, R, (2009) Emotion Regulation: aggression, ADHD and violence in families In. Dallos.R and Vetere, A. *Systemic Therapy and Attachment Narratives,* London: Routledge.

Dallos, R. (2006) Attachment Narrative Therapy. Maidenhead: Open University Dallos, R. and Vetere, A. (2005) *Research Methods in Psychotherapy* , Maidenhead : McGraw –Hill/Open Univ. Press Press/McGraw Hill.

Dallos, R. and Denford, S. (2008) A qualitative exploration of relationship and attachment themes in families with an eating disorder. *Clinical Child Psychology and Psychiatry.* 13: 305-322 Dow, J. (1996) Family Therapy and ADHD. *Family Therapy News, p.14.*

Erdman, P. (1998) Conceptualising ADHD as a contextual response to parental attachment. *The American Journal of Family Therapy,* 26: 177 - 185.

Finzi -Dottan, R. Manor, I. and Tyano, S. (2006) ADHD, temperament and parental styles as predictors of the child's attachment patterns. *Child Psychiatry and Human Development,* 37(2) :103 -114.

Farnfield, S., Hautamäki, A., Nørbech, P. and Sahhar, N., (2010) DMM Assessments of Attachment and Adaptation: Procedures, Validity, and Utility . *Clinical Child Psychology and Psychiatry,* (Special Issue - ..Attachment, Children and Families: The Dynamic-Maturational-Model). 15(3): 313-328).

George, C., Kaplan, N., and Main, M. (1986, 1996). Adult Attachment Interview. Unpublished manuscript. University of California, Berkeley.

George, C. Kaplan, N. and Main, M. (1985) The Berkeley Adult Attachment Interview. Unpublished Protocol. Dept. of Psychology, University of California, Berkeley CA.

Gergen, K. (1999) An Invitation to Social Constructionism. London: Sage

Kozlowska, K. and Foley, S. and Crittenden, P. (2006) Factitious Illness by Proxy: Understanding Underlying Psychological Processes and Motivations. *ANJF.* 27(2) : 92-104.

Kissgen, R.,Krischer, M. , Kummetat, V., Spiess, R., Schleiffer, R. And Sevecke, K (2009) Attachment representation in mothers of children with attention deficit hyperactive disorder. *Psychopathology*, 43(3) : 201- 2008.

Ladnier, R.D. and Massanari, A.E. (2000) Treating ADHD as attention deficit hyperactive disorder. In T.M. Levy *Handbook of Attachment Interventions* (pp27-65. San Diego: Academic Press).

Liotti, G. (2004) Trauma, dissociation and Disorganised Attachments: Three strands of a single braid. *Psychotherapy: Theory ,Research Practice and* Training. 41: 472-486.

Main, K., Kaplan, N. and Cassidy, J. (1985) 'Security in infancy, childhood, and adulthood: a move to the level of representation'. In I. Bretherton and

E. Water (eds), *Monographs of the Society for Research and Child Development,* Serial No. 209.50: Nos1-2. Chicago: the University of Chicago Press.

Mash, E.J and Johnson, C. (2005) ADHD and the family: A developmental psychopathology perspective. In. J.L. Hudson and R.M.Rapee (eds) *Psychopathology and the family,* New York: Elsever Science.

Mikulincer, M. and Shaver, P.R. (2007) *Attachment in Adulthood: Structure, dynamics and change,* New York: Guilford Press.

Moretti, M.M, Holland, R. And Peterson, S. (1994) Long term outcome of an attachment – based program for conduct disorder. *Canadian Journal of Psychiatry,* 39:360 – 370.

NICE(2006) National Institute for Health and Clinical Excellence, ADHD : a draft scope for consultation. http:/www.nice.orgsa.uk.

Nylund, D. (2000) Treating Huckleberry Finn. San Fransisco: Jossey – Bass

Ringer, R. and Crittenden, P.M. (2006) Eating disorders and attachment: The effects of hidden family processes on eating disorders. *European Eating Disorders Review.* 14. 1- 12.

Robson, C. (2002) *Real World Research.* Oxford: Blackwell.

Scharfstein, S. (2006) Task Force on the Effects of Violence on Children. Washington, USA: American Psychiatric Association.

Schore, A (1994) Affect Regulation and the Origin of the Self. Hillsdale, New Jersey: Erlbaum.

Vetere, A. and Cooper, J. (2006) The effects of domestic violence on children: trauma, resilience and breaking the cycle of violence. *The Journal of Critical Psychology.*

In: ADHD
Editors: R. Thompson and N. J. Miller
ISBN: 978-1-62417-107-9

Chapter 3

DO PROFESSIONS DIFFER IN THEIR BELIEFS ABOUT THE CAUSES AND TREATMENT OF ATTENTION-DEFICIT HYPERACTIVITY DISORDER?

Rachel Dryer, Michael J. Kiernan and Graham A. Tyson
School of Psychology, Charles Sturt University,
Bathurst, New South Wales, Australia

ABSTRACT

Key health organisations in Western countries, such as the National Institute for Health and Clinical Excellence (2008) in the United Kingdom, and more recently, the American Academy of Paediatrics (2011) in the United States, have advocated multimodal and multidisciplinary approaches to the diagnosis and treatment of Attention-deficit hyperactivity disorder (ADHD). However, despite these clinical best practice guidelines, there is little evidence of a general adoption of interdisciplinary collaboration and practice. One impediment to the implementation of multidisciplinary practice may be the beliefs that different professionals (and professional bodies) hold about the causes and treatment of ADHD. This chapter reviews the results of research that examined the beliefs of professional groups engaged in the diagnosis and treatment of ADHD about (i) the causes of ADHD and (ii) the efficacy of general treatment approaches. Following the review, other possible impediments to the adoption of interdisciplinary collaboration and practice are also discussed.

Attention-deficit hyperactivity disorder (ADHD) is currently conceptualised as a neurobehavioral condition that is characterised by developmentally inappropriate levels of inattention, impulsivity and motor overactivity (American Psychiatric Association [APA], 2000). It is estimated to be present in 3% to 7% of the school-aged population and can result in significant impairment in academic, social and family functioning (APA, 2000, Barkley, 2006). While the symptoms of hyperactivity, impulsivity and inattention may decline with age, up to 90% of adolescents with ADHD continue to struggle with this condition and remain functionally impaired in early adulthood (Beiderman, Mick and Faraone, 2000). As adults, these individuals are more likely to be involved in teen pregnancy, sexually transmitted diseases, and motor-vehicle accidents and to experience depression (Barkley, 2002).

Given the prevalence and serious consequences of ADHD, an enormous body of research has been conducted into both its aetiology and treatment. However, these two key facets of ADHD remain controversial for both the families and professionals involved (Barkley, 2006; Golman, Genel, Bezman and Stanelz, 1998; Brimble, 2009; Jensen, 2000; Kewley, 2001; Thapar, Holmes, Poulton and Harrington, 1999). This controversy has led to organisations such as the `National Institute for Health and Clinical Excellence' (NICE, 2008), and the American Academy of Paediatrics (AAP, 2011) to develop clinical practice guidelines for the identification and treatment or management of this condition. Both of these guidelines advocate a multidisciplinary approach to ADHD and recommend better integration of medical and mental health services for individuals with ADHD and their families. For example, the NICE guidelines recommend the formation of multidisciplinary specialist ADHD teams and/or clinics to provide diagnostic, treatment and consultation services. These specialist teams would also be involved in implementing systems of communication and protocols for information sharing among professionals within the paediatric, child and adolescent, forensic, and adult mental health services. The NICE guidelines further recommend the formation of multi-agency groups comprised of representatives from the multidisciplinary specialist ADHD team, paediatrics, mental health and learning disability services, forensic services, education and social services, and parent support groups. These multi-agency groups would, among other functions, oversee the implementation of the NICE guidelines, and the provision of ADHD education and training programs for both professionals and families involved. In recognition of the complex nature of ADHD and its co-morbidity with other conditions, the NICE guidelines state that the diagnosis should be made on the basis of a comprehensive clinical and psychosocial assessment, a comprehensive developmental and psychiatric history and observer assessment of the person's mental state. For children and adolescents, an assessment of their parents' or caregivers' mental health should also be undertaken. Consequently, the evaluation for a diagnosis of ADHD can involve referrals to health, education and social care professionals (e.g., general practitioners, child psychiatrists, paediatricians, child/school psychologists, social workers and adult mental health professionals). Furthermore, unlike previous NICE guidelines, the current guidelines state that behavioural therapies, rather than medication, should be the first-line treatment for pre-school and school-aged children and adolescents. These behavioural therapies include parent-training/education programs, behavioural interventions in the classroom, cognitive behavioural therapy (CBT) and/or social skills training (NICE, 2008). These therapeutic approaches are usually implemented in the home and school settings by parents and teachers respectively. However, the implementation of these interventions can also involve other professionals such as child/school psychologists and social workers who deliver the guidance and training in specific behaviour modification principles and techniques. Consequently, successful implementation of these first-line treatment/management approaches requires greater consultation and collaboration across the different disciplines involved in the care of the child diagnosed with ADHD.

Similar to the NICE guidelines, the current AAP clinical practice guidelines (2011) promote the development of alliances between medical and non-medical professionals in assisting children with ADHD and their families. As in the previous 2000 guidelines, the current AAP guidelines recommend that during the process of diagnosing ADHD, the paediatrician should consult the Diagnostic and Statistical Manual of Mental Disorders (currently the DSM-IV-TR [Text Revision]). This recommendation is made partly on the basis that the DSM-IV-TR is used by professionals in psychiatry, psychology, health care systems, and primary care and would therefore assist in facilitating better communication between the different professions involved. In contrast to the previous guidelines, the current guidelines now specifically recommend obtaining additional information from parents/caregivers, teachers, and other school and mental health clinicians during the diagnostic process. In diagnosing ADHD, the current guidelines further recommend that an assessment be conducted by other specialists (e.g., child psychiatrists, developmental-behavioural paediatricians, neurodevelopmental disability physicians, child neurologists and child or school psychologists) to identify or exclude co-existing conditions. The guidelines' promotion of multidisciplinary collaboration can further be found in their recommendation for treatment and management. In order to effectively deliver the required on-going care for children with ADHD, the guidelines recommend the establishment of bidirectional communication with teachers and other school and mental health clinicians involved in the child's care. Consistent with the NICE guidelines, the current AAP guidelines recommend the application of evidence-based behaviour therapy as the first-line treatment, but only for preschool-aged children. In contrast to the NICE guidelines, pharmacotherapy is the recommended first-line treatment for school-aged children and adolescents, with behavioural therapies recommended only as a concurrent treatment for these age-groups. Despite these differences in treatment recommendations, both sets of clinical guidelines require greater involvement of non-medical professionals (e.g., education and mental health services) in the diagnosis and treatment of ADHD.

The NICE and AAP clinical practice guidelines recognise the essential contribution of professionals from discipline groups other than the medical profession in addressing ADHD. However, the available data suggest that there is little interaction between the various professions, especially between medical practitioners and other mental health professionals, when diagnosing and treating ADHD. For example, Kwasman, Tinsley and Lepper (1995) surveyed 380 paediatricians in the US, and reported that only 39.1% had obtained information from the school attended by the child diagnosed with ADHD; only 18.7% were likely to refer children with ADHD to other professionals such as psychologists, special educators, social workers, or some other professional in a related discipline; and only 14.6% reported that their patients consulted a psychologist before beginning treatment on stimulant medication. This low level of interdisciplinary interaction reported by Kwasman, et al may, in part, be due to the study being conducted prior to the 2001 publication of the first edition of the AAP ADHD guidelines.

The impact of the AAP clinical practice guidelines, particularly on interdisciplinary interaction and collaboration in the diagnosis of ADHD was examined by Rushton, Fant and Clark (2004) who surveyed 723 primary care medical practitioners in the US about their adherence to these guidelines. They reported that many of the respondents were familiar with the AAP guidelines and had adopted many aspects of the guidelines' recommendations into their practice. Specifically, in comparison to Kwasman et al. (1995), Rushton et al. found an increase in the level of interaction between medical practitioners and teachers such that approximately 78% of the medical practitioners obtained information from schools using teacher rating scales to assist them in the diagnosis of ADHD. However, only 17.3% of respondents indicated that they routinely referred their patients to other professionals (e.g., psychologists, social workers, or psychiatrist) for initial ADHD evaluation and diagnosis.

The impact of the 2001 AAP guidelines along with other AAP initiatives (e.g., ADHD toolkits, online CME module [www.eqipp.org]) on attitudes and practices of paediatricians was also evaluated by Wolraich, Bard, Stein, Rushton and O'Connor (2010) who surveyed AAP members in 1999 ($N = 452$) and again in 2005 ($N = 551$). They reported an increase in the routine use of parent and teacher behaviour rating scales in the assessment for ADHD over time, but also reported a significant decline from 27% to 21% in the frequency of use of psychoeducational testing in the diagnostic process. Less than 14 percent of respondents in either survey indicated that they routinely used neuropsychological testing in their evaluation for ADHD. With regards to treatment practices, three quarters of the respondents in both surveys indicated that they frequently or always recommended classroom evaluation and modification. Interestingly, while more paediatricians in the 2005 survey compared to the 1999 survey indicated that they provided parents with information about appropriate parenting skills, only a very small proportion (approximately 10%) indicated that they referred parents to a formal parent training group outside of their practice. In addition, less than 10% of those who completed the 2005 survey indicated that they would frequently or always refer their patients to alternative (complementary) therapies. These results suggest that while there has been an increase in the level of interaction between medical practitioners and teachers as a result of the AAP guidelines (2000, 2001), the level of interaction between medical practitioners and other professionals (especially mental health clinicians) remain very limited.

Adherence to the multidisciplinary approach recommended by the NICE and AAP clinical practice guidelines assumes that the professionals involved in the assessment and treatment of ADHD have common beliefs about the condition. The low level of inter-disciplinary interaction reported in the literature may, in part, be due to differences in beliefs about the aetiology and treatment of ADHD held by the various professional groups. Personal beliefs about the causes of a problem, its expected course and prognosis are sometimes referred to as an implicit theory or explanatory model and they evolve from the individual's personal experiences and their social and cultural environment (Furnham, 1988). For professional groups, beliefs about disorders/conditions would also be mediated by their professional training and the views promoted by their relevant professional associations (e.g., AAP, American Psychiatric Association, American Psychological Association). These personal beliefs serve as a guide to interpersonal behaviour and would influence the holder's responses to individuals with that problem/condition. The study of implicit theories has been used to understand how various sections of the population understand behaviours and conditions such as bulimia nervosa (Dryer, Tyson and Kiernan, in press), juvenile delinquency (Tyson and Hubert, 2000), depression (Furnham and Kuyken, 1991) and schizophrenia (Furnham and Bower, 1992). Furthermore, members of different professional groups can hold implicit theories that vary according to their professional background and training (Kuyken, Brewin, Power and Furnham, 1992; Masse, Couture and Anciaux, 2010; Roskin, Carsen, Rabiner and Marell, 1988).

There has been limited examination of the implicit theories of ADHD held by professionals engaged in the diagnosis and treatment of ADHD. Most of the studies that have explored professional beliefs and attitudes of ADHD have focused on single disciplines. For example, Shaw, Wagner, Eastwood and Mitchell (2003) conducted a qualitative study on the attitudes and practices of 28 Australian general medical practitioners with regards to the diagnosis and management of this condition. Many of the medical practitioners surveyed attribute ADHD to external factors such as parenting style/management, and social and environmental stressors (e.g., family dysfunction). Most also believed that ADHD was over-diagnosed as a result of medical labels being applied to variations in normal behaviour or medicalising a social problem caused by ineffective parenting. Other causal factors such as being exposed to violence on television and dietary hypersensitivity were not regarded as being as important to causes related to the family unit and parenting style. Despite many of the general medical practitioners attributing ADHD to normative social factors, the majority of these practitioners did not refer clients to non-medical professionals (e.g., psychologists, social workers). Instead the majority referred their clients to medical specialists such as paediatricians and psychiatrists. This low rate of referrals to non-medical professionals is consistent with the low interdisciplinary interaction between medical and non-medical practitioners reported in the literature. While Eastwood and Mitchell study does provide some insights into the beliefs and attitudes of medical practitioners, it is limited by its small sample size.

Relatively more research has been conducted exploring teachers' beliefs regarding the cause and treatment for ADHD. For example, DiBattista and Shepherd (1993) surveyed 389 teachers in Canada with regards to their beliefs concerning the effects of sugar and other commonly consumed food items on the behaviour of both hyperactive and normal (i.e., nonhyperactive) children. They found that more than 80% of the teachers believed that sugar consumption adversely affected the behaviour of normal and hyperactive children. Furthermore, more than 65% of these teachers reported making recommendations to parents to reduce their child's sugar intake as a way of controlling their child's activity levels. Jerome, Gordon and Hustler (1995) examined the knowledge and attitudes of 439 American and 350 Canadian teachers regarding this condition and found that these teachers regarded ADHD as a valid clinical syndrome. However, despite having a good knowledge base regarding the aetiology and educational implications of this condition, many endorsed the effectiveness of strategies involving dietary changes as an effective way of addressing this condition. Furthermore, only 14% of these teachers had been involved in the diagnosis and management of this condition by outside professionals. More recently, Weyandt, Fulton, Schepman, Verdi and Wilson (2009) examined teacher and school psychologist knowledge of ADHD using the 'ADHD Beliefs Scale' (Johnston and Freeman, 2002). This scale consisted of 24 statements regarding the possible causes of ADHD and appropriate treatment options, for which respondents were required to indicate their level of endorsement for each statement. Respondents comprised 42 general classroom teachers, 36 special education teachers and 54 school psychologists. Responses to the 'ADHD Beliefs Scale' were scored using two subscales labelled as 'reasonable beliefs' and 'false belief'. The 'reasonable beliefs' subscale was comprised of beliefs that have been supported by the scientific literature whereas; the 'false belief' subscale was comprised of beliefs that had not been validated in the literature. Weyandt et al., reported that in both groups of teachers, knowledge of ADHD appeared to be limited. While the special education teachers provided stronger endorsement for items on the 'reasonable beliefs' subscale than on the 'false belief' subscale, general classroom teachers showed the opposite pattern of endorsement. Furthermore, both groups of teachers provided strong endorsement for the statement, "Special diets are effective treatments for ADHD" and 28% of general classroom teachers also endorsed the item of "Vitamin therapy may effectively treat the symptoms of ADHD". These findings are consistent with those reported in previous studies indicating that teachers generally believe in the effectiveness of dietary treatment approaches for this condition. In contrast, school psychologists compared to teachers, scored significantly higher on the 'reasonable beliefs' subscale and significantly lower on the 'false belief' subscale. However, examination of individual items suggested a lack of certainty in endorsing statements such as "Individual child therapy is an effective treatment for ADHD" and "Children with ADHD inherit the disorder from someone in the family" which Weyandt et al., identify as reasonable belief options for ADHD.

While the studies described above give some idea of the implicit theories of ADHD held by those in specific professions, none of them address the issue of possible differences between professions. One of the few studies that have explored this issue across multiple disciplines is Hughes (1999) who questioned nine health professionals from the disciplines of paediatrics, neuropsychiatry, psychiatry and educational psychology regarding their beliefs of the cause and treatment of ADHD. Eight of the nine participants attributed this condition to a biological cause while seven identified the home environment as an additional causal factor. Three of the participants were sceptical of ADHD existing as a valid clinical syndrome. All of the participants endorsed the use of medication in addressing ADHD, while four of the participants also advocated the need for behaviour management in the school setting. Only one participant identified making dietary changes an important strategy for addressing this condition. While Hughes' study provides some interesting insights, the methodology and small sample size make it difficult to generalise the results. In an effort to more systematically examine the implicit theories of professional groups engaged in the diagnosis and treatment of ADHD, we carried out two studies. The first study reported the results of a survey of 494 medical and nonmedical professionals about their beliefs about the causes of ADHD (Dryer, Kiernan and Tyson, 2006a) and the efficacy of various treatment strategies for this condition (Dryer, Kiernan and Tyson, 2012). The medical practitioners comprised general medical practitioners (N = 82) and paediatricians (N = 22), while the nonmedical professionals were comprised of psychologists (N = 101), occupational therapists (N = 63), social workers (N = 71), dieticians (N = 20), and primary school teachers (N = 135). These professional groups were selected because within the Australian health system they are potentially able to be consulted about ADHD, or referred clients with this condition. The survey questionnaire required participants to rate 46 causal explanations and 23 treatment /management strategies for this condition. These questionnaire items were generated from a pilot study involving 25 participants in the targeted professions. Participants' beliefs were assessed on a 5-point rating scale (causal factors, 0 = unimportant, 4 = extremely important; treatment /management, 0 = not at all effective, 4 = extremely effective). Further details of the questionnaire and its construction can be found in Dryer, Kiernan and Tyson (2006a).

Principle component analyses, conducted on obtained ratings for the items, identified six causal factors. The six causal factors were labelled *Home Environment* (i.e., items loading on this factor related to an unstable home environment and poor parenting style), *School Environment* (i.e., child's difficulty adjusting to school work and the school environment), *Toxins* (i.e., chemical exposure in utero or through diet), *Brain Damage* (i.e., brain damage, birth complications and developmental delay), *Brain Function* (i.e., chemical imbalance in the brain, brain dysfunction, genetic predisposition), and *Psychological Problems* (i.e., anxiety and depression). Both parental and professional groups provided the strongest endorsement for the *Brain Function* factor, suggesting that all the groups regarded ADHD as having neurological and genetic causes. For the group as a whole, there were no significant differences in the endorsement of the *Home Environment*, *School Environment*, *Brain Damage* and *Psychological Problems* factors. However, endorsement for the *Toxins* factor was found to be significantly lower compared to the level of endorsement for the factors of *School Environment*, *Brain Damage* and *Psychological Problems*.

Interestingly, the medical and non-medical professionals were found to hold relatively similar beliefs about the causal factors of ADHD. The professional groups did not significantly differ in their endorsement of the *School Environment*, *Brain Function*, *Brain Damage* and *Psychological Problems* factors as potential causes. The only difference observed between the professions was on the *Toxins* factor, where primary school teachers were found to attribute more importance to causes related to teratogens and toxins as a cause of ADHD compared to paediatricians and general practitioners. This finding is consistent with results of previous studies that have reported that teachers believe that ADHD can be caused by changes in the diet or excessive consumption of sugar (e.g., Barbaresi and Olsen, 1998; DiBattista and Sheperd, 1993; Ghanizadeh, Bahredar and Moeini, 2006; Jerome, Gordon and Hustler, 1994).

With regards to beliefs about the efficacy of various treatment strategies for ADHD, the four treatment factors identified using principle component analysis, were labelled *Non-traditional Interventions* (i.e., dietary changes, sound therapy, biofeedback, kinesiology and chiropractic manipulations), *Parent Interventions* (i.e., parent training and input), *School-based Interventions* (i.e., changes to the educational structure, increased teacher support and input), and *Medical and Allied Health Interventions* (i.e., medication, occupational therapy, speech therapy and providing a structured environment). The strategies contained within the *School-based Interventions* factor were clearly regarded by both parents and professionals to be the most effective treatment approach to ADHD. The next groups of strategies to be considered to be effective were those contained within the factors of *Parent Interventions* and the *Medical and Allied Health Interventions*. The strategies regarded to be least effective were those contained within the *Non-traditional Interventions* factor. This factor received a significantly lower level of endorsement compared to the other three treatment factors, with a mean factor score reflecting a "not at all effective" response.

As indicated above, there was a high degree of agreement between the professional groups with regard to their endorsement of the treatment /management factors. The only exception to this general concordance was in the primary school teacher's endorsement of the *Parent Interventions* factor. Primary school teachers, compared to the other groups in this study, were found to provide stronger endorsement for strategies involving parents. One possible explanation for this difference is that primary school teachers are likely to be involved in daily interactions with children with ADHD and their families. They would also have first-hand experience of the difficulties associated with implementing treatment strategies in the school setting and may be more aware of the limitations of such approaches, compared to the other professionals. Consequently, they may have a better appreciation of the need to implement treatment strategies in both the home and school settings.

Teachers did not endorse the *Non-traditional Interventions* factor higher than the other professional groups. This was unexpected as some previous studies (e.g., DiBattista and Shepherd, 1993; Weyandt, et al., 2009) have shown that teachers indicated strong support for the use of health food supplements (e.g., vitamins and fatty acids) and dietary changes involving elimination of food additives or those that cause allergies. One explanation for the lack of difference between the groups is that the belief factor contained both non-dietary (e.g., sound therapy and biofeedback) and dietary treatment strategies for ADHD. Thus to explore whether teachers, relative to other professionals, provided stronger endorsement for strategies involving dietary changes, the mean level of endorsement for the three diet related items within this factor was examined. This analysis did reveal a significant difference between teachers and the professional groups of medical practitioners and psychologists, with teachers providing stronger endorsement for treatment strategies involving dietary changes.

Interestingly, the Dryer, Kiernan and Tyson (2012) study found relatively strong endorsement by both medical and nonmedical professionals for the use of medication in the treatment of ADHD. The level of endorsement for this single item indicated that the respondents on average considered medication to be effective (i.e., mean rating = 3.00, *SD* = 1.01). The medication item was one of the ten most endorsed treatment strategies. This suggests that the low levels of interdisciplinary interaction reported in the literature are unlikely to be due to differences amongst medical and non-medical professionals in their beliefs about the use of psycho-stimulant medication and other pharmacotherapy.

A limitation in the Dryer, Kiernan and Tyson (2006a; 2012) study was that it did not examine whether the respondents accepted ADHD as a valid clinical syndrome. One could argue that the presence or absence of a diagnostic label can influence beliefs about the causes of the observed behaviours and may have follow-on consequences with regards to decisions made about treatment. To address this issue, we examined the impact of diagnostic labelling on professional's causal explanations and decisions regarding treatment in a vignette study that manipulated the presence versus absence of the label 'ADHD' (Dryer, Kiernan and Tyson, 2006b). One of two versions of a vignette was presented to 487 nonmedical professionals (i.e., psychologists, primary school teachers, dieticians and occupational therapists). The vignette described a child exhibiting the symptoms associated with ADHD, with one version including containing the phrase 'recently diagnosed with ADHD' while the other contained no reference to ADHD. After reading the vignette, the professionals completed a questionnaire examining their beliefs about the causes of ADHD and its treatment and management. This questionnaire was developed based on the results obtained from the Dryer, Kiernan and Tyson, (2006a; 2012) study. The professionals were required to indicate their level of endorsement for each item using a 5-point rating scale (causes: 0 = unimportant, 4 = extremely important; treatment: 0 = not at all effective, 4 = extremely effective). The questionnaire responses were scored according to the factor groupings (i.e., six causal factors, four treatment factors) identified previously. This study found that the inclusion of the ADHD label changed the causal explanations for the behaviours described in the vignette but not their beliefs about the efficacy of treatment approaches for this condition. The presence of the ADHD diagnostic label resulted in professionals providing stronger endorsement for neurological or genetic causes for this condition (i.e., the *Brain Function* factor). In contrast, absence of the diagnostic label resulted in stronger endorsement of causes associated with parenting style and the home environment (i.e., the *Home Environment* factor). This finding indicates that when the same behaviours of inattention, impulsivity and hyperactivity are presented to professionals with the diagnostic label of 'ADHD', they are more likely to assume the existence of an underlying physical or biological condition. Consequently, these professionals may be less inclined to look for social, environmental or psychological causes for the observed behaviours. Despite this, , however, the presence of a diagnostic label did not change the professionals' beliefs about how best to treat the behaviours of inattention, impulsivity and hyperactivity associated with this condition. The inclusion of the ADHD label did not lead to a greater endorsement of medical and allied health treatment strategies. Instead, intervention strategies involving teachers and schools (i.e., *School-based Intervention* factor) were the preferred approach by the professionals regardless of whether the behaviours were described as ADHD or not.

The results of our studies indicate a high degree of agreement between the professional groups with regard to their causal explanations for ADHD and their beliefs about the effectiveness of various treatment strategies for this condition. Furthermore, the professional beliefs about treatment strategies are relatively consistent with the recommendations outlined in the NICE (2008) and AAP (2011) clinical practice guidelines (i.e., the combined use of medication as well as strategies that involve parent-training/education and interventions implemented by teachers in the classroom). Therefore, the low level of interdisciplinary interaction and collaboration that has been reported in the literature is unlikely to be due to differences in beliefs held by the various professionals. However, the question of why there is an underutilisation of multidisciplinary approaches remains. One possible contributing factor to the low interdisciplinary interaction and collaboration is the cost effectiveness of these treatment approaches. The landmark Multimodal Treatment Study for Children with ADHD (MTA) (MTA Cooperative Group, 1999; 2004) found that children diagnosed with ADHD who received a combined (multimodal) treatment program involving medication and behavioural interventions (parent training, behavioural support for teachers, social skills training) showed greater symptom alleviation at both 14 months and 24 months of treatment than those treated with other approaches. However, the combined treatment was not significantly better than medication alone on most treatment indices. Both the combined and medication alone treatments were superior to the behavioural interventions alone, and all interventions were found to be better than a community treatment control condition, although even here improvements were reported. Thus, while the combined (multi-modal) treatment were shown to be the most efficacious treatment, it can be argued that the small additional gains observed for this relatively more expensive treatment approach need to be weighed against alternative, less expensive, approaches.

The full cost of untreated ADHD for the individual, families, schools and for the wider community is difficult to assess. However, the costs associated with ADHD are likely to be as high, if not higher, than that of medical conditions (e.g., asthma) and childhood mental health problems (Pelham, Foster and Robb, 2007). Studies examining the cost-effectiveness of ADHD interventions, therefore, need to examine variables such as the effectiveness of interventions in alleviating the long-term cost to the community, the long-term effectiveness of treatment given the unit (i.e., session) costs and treatment duration, and the estimated gains obtained by one approach over and above others (such as the MTA combined treatment over medication alone). In the light of these considerations, Foster et al. (2007) re-analysed the MTA data in relation to the cost of the treatment conditions relative to the reported treatment gains. They concluded that the combined treatment approach was more cost-effective only when comorbid conditions were an issue for the client; otherwise, the most cost-effective intervention for the core ADHD symptoms was medication alone. In the light of these results, and given the difficulty in estimating the actual long-term personal and community cost of more complex presentations of ADHD it could be argued that it is reasonable for health services to opt for the most cost effective treatment for the majority of clients, which is management by medication only.

The use of the treatment approach that is perceived to be most cost-effective, impacts upon parental options and choices. Irrespective of parents' own beliefs and attitudes to the treatment of ADHD, they are dependent upon the treatment options available and, in most cases; medication management is likely to be the only available option. In fact, medication, as a treatment option, is made even cheaper in some countries by the availability of subsidies for the cost of stimulant medication (e.g., Australian Government: Department of Health and Ageing, 2007). Thus, despite the congruence of beliefs about the nature and treatment of ADHD held by a wide range of professional groups, the establishment of multidisciplinary treatment teams is unlikely to occur where service delivery planning is dependent upon decisions about the cost-effectiveness of treatment options.

Another financial barrier to providing multidisciplinary treatment approaches is that current reimbursement practices are largely limited to face-to-face visits (Brinkman and Epstein, 2011). Multimodal treatment approaches to ADHD require a level of infrastructure to support the care coordination of the client by multiple professionals and to facilitate communication between all members of the care team. Brinkman and Epstein (2011), in their review of evidence-based guidelines for the treatment of ADHD, argue that these reimbursement practices create difficulties in sustaining aspects of multimodal treatments that exists outside of face-to-face visits (e.g., sessions with parents without the ADHD client being present, treatment planning and treatment team meetings that may not include the ADHD client, or at times even family members) and to support the infrastructure that is needed to deliver these treatment approaches.

Other barriers to the delivery of multimodal treatment approaches identified by Brinkman and Epstein (2011) include medical practitioners not having a prominent role in the delivery of behavioural therapies and encountering difficulties in accessing behaviour therapy services for their client from the educational and mental health sectors. Lack of accessible paediatric mental health services, quality of available therapists, long waiting lists and inadequate medical insurance coverage have also been identifies as some of the factors that prevented medical practitioners from recommending psychosocial therapies to their client (Reeves and Anthony, 2009; Rushton, Fant and Clark, 2004).

Cost effectiveness and resource/financial restrictions are unlikely to be the only barriers to the development and adoption of multidisciplinary treatment approaches as advocated in the NICE (2008) and AAP (2011) guidelines. A more fundamental issue may be that professionals are unfamiliar with the guidelines. A study by Shaw, Mitchell, Wagner and Eastwood (2002) of the attitudes and practices of Australian general medical practitioners found a reluctance on their part to play any role in the management of this condition due, in part, to unfamiliarity with the guidelines of the time. A more recent qualitative study conducted by Bailey and Simpson (2008) of professionals involved in ADHD treatment in the UK found that many of those interviewed reported that they had either not heard of the NICE guidelines, or had heard of them, but reported not reading them. Bailey and Simpson also reported that some of the professionals who were familiar with the guidelines rejected them as being "too medical" and of limited usefulness or applicability to their own practice. Furthermore, while there was a consensus amongst the professionals that the treatment for ADHD should be multimodal in nature, the non-medical clinicians rejected the NICE guidelines as it was perceived to advocate a medical framework for the diagnosis and treatment of this condition. When combined with the results of our studies, it suggests that even though beliefs held by the various professionals about ADHD are not significantly divergent, tensions exist amongst some professionals with regard to the 'medicalisation' of this condition. Such tensions may be contributing to the low interdisciplinary interaction between professionals and to the underutilisation of multidisciplinary treatment approaches.

To conclude, while there is a general recommendation for a multi-disciplinary assessment and interventions for ADHD, there has been a low take-up of this recommendation. This chapter shows that the low take-up is unlikely to be due to differences in the attitudes and beliefs of health professionals and teachers about the causes and treatment of this condition, but is more likely to be related to policy decisions of health services and governments about the cost-effectiveness of treatment options. Specifically, as medication management appears to be the most cost-effective treatment approach for most children with ADHD, at least in the short-term, and in the absence of reliable methods of assessing the life-time cost of the condition for the community, medication only options are likely to continue to be the funded treatment option, This in turn, will drive professional practice and parental choice.

About the Authors

Rachel Dryer, PhD, is a lecturer in the School of Psychology at Charles Sturt University. Her research interests are in the areas of developmental conditions. Her research projects reflect an interest in examining not only a range of theoretical and applied questions but also clinical and social issues.

Michael J. Kiernan, PhD, is an Associate Professor of Clinical Psychology. He is head of the School of Psychology at Charles Sturt University. He has clinical and research interests in developmental conditions.

Graham A. Tyson, PhD, is an Associate Professor of Psychology at Charles Sturt University. He is a social psychologist, and his research interests include social cognition and social justice issues.

REFERENCES

American Academy of Pediatrics (2011). ADHD: Clinical practice guidelines for the diagnosis, evaluation, and treatment of attention-deficit/hyperactive disorder in children and adolescents. *Pediatrics*, *128* (5), 1007-1022.

American Psychiatric Association (2000). *Diagnostic and statistical manual of mental disorders* (4th ed., text rev.). Washington, DC: Author.

Australian Government: Department of Health and Ageing (2007). Pharmaceutical benefits scheme – listing of Strattera (atomoxetine). Retrieved from http://www.health.gov.au/internet/budget/publishing.nsf/Content/budget2007-hfact13.htm

Barkley, R. A. (2006). *Attention-deficit hyperactivity disorder: A handbook for diagnosis and treatment* (3rd ed.). New York, NY: Guilford Press.

Barkely, R. A. (2002). International consensus statement on ADHD. *Clinical Child and Family Psychology Review*, *5* (2), 89-111.

Bailey, S., and Simpson, A. (2008). Attitudes towards attention deficit hyperactivity disorder in child and adolescent mental health service teams. *Mental Health Practice, 11(10),* 26-31.

Beiderman, J., Mick, E., and Faraone, S. V. (2000). Age-dependent decline of symptoms of attention deficit hyperactivity disorder: impact of remission definition and symptom type. *American Journal of Psychiatry*, *157*(5), 816-818.

Brimble, M. J. (2009). Diagnosis and management of ADHD: a new way forward? *Community Practitioner*, *82* (10), 34-37.

Brinkman, W. B., and and Epstein, J. N. (2011). Promoting productive interactions between parents and physicians in the treatment of children with attention-deficit/hyperactivity disorder. *Expert Review of Neurotherapeutics*, *11* (4), 579-588.

DiBattista, D., and Shepherd, M. (1993). Primary school teachers' beliefs and advice to parents concerning sugar consumption and activity in children. *Psychological Reports*, *72*, 47-55.

Dryer, R., Kiernan, M.J., and Tyson, G.A. (2006a). Implicit theories of the characteristics and causes of attention-deficit hyperactivity disorder held by parents and professionals in the psychological, educational, medical and allied health fields. *Australian Journal of Psychology*, *58* (2), 79-92.

Dryer, R., Kiernan, M.J., and Tyson, G.A. (2006b). The effects of Diagnostic labelling on the implicit theories of attention-deficit/hyperactivity disorder held by health professionals. *Behaviour Change*, *23* (3), 177-185.

Dryer, R., Kiernan, M.J., and Tyson, G.A. (2012). Parental and professional beliefs on the treatment and management of ADHD. *Journal of Attention Disorders, 16* (5),398-405.

Dryer, R., Tyson, G.A., and Kiernan, M.J. (in press). Bulimia nervosa: Professional and lay people's beliefs about the causes. *Australian Psychologist.*

Foster, E.M., Jensen, P.S., Schlander, M., Pelham, W.E., Hechtman, L., Arnold, L.E., Swanson, J.M. and Wigal, T. (2007). Treatment for ADHD: Is more complex treatment cost-effective for more complex cases? *Health Services Research, 42,*165-182.

Furnham, A. (1988). *Lay theories: Everyday understanding of problems in the social sciences.* Oxford: Pergamon Press.

Furnham, A., and Bower, P. (1992). A comparison of academic and lay theories of schizophrenia. *British Journal of Psychiatry, 161*, 201-210.

Furnham, A., and Kuyken, W. (1991). Lay theories of depression. *Journal of Social Behavior and Personality, 6*, 329-342.

Goldman, L. S., Genel, M., Bezman, R.J., and Stanelz, P. J. (1998). Diagnosis and treatment of attention-deficit/hyperactivity disorder in children and adolescents. *Journal of American Medical Association, 279* (14), 1100-1107.

Hughes, L. A. (2000) How the Professions Perceive AD/HD. In: Cooper, P., and Bilton, K. (Eds) *ADHD Research, Practice and Opinion.* pp. 187-202. London: Whurr publication.

Jensen, P.S. (2000). Current concepts and controversies in the diagnosis and treatment of attention deficit hyperactivity disorder. *Current Psychiatry Reports, 2* (2), 102-109.

Jerome, L., Gordon, M., and Hustler, P. (1994). A comparison of American and Canadian teachers' knowledge and attitudes towards attention deficit hyperactivity disorder (ADHD). *The Canadian Journal of Psychiatry, 39* (9), 563-567.

Johnston, C., and Freeman, W.S. (2002). Parents' beliefs about ADHD: Implications for assessment and treatment. *The ADHD Report, 10*, 6-9.

Kewley, G. (2001). ADHD: *Recognition reality and resolution.* Melbourne, Australia: Acer Press.

Kuyken, W., Brewin, C.R., Power, M.J., and Furnham, A. (1992). Causal beliefs about depression in depressed patients, clinical psychologists and lay persons. *British Journal of Medical Psychology, 65*, 257-268.

Kwasman, A., Tinsley, B. J., and Lepper, H.S. (1995). Pediatrician's knowledge and attitudes concerning diagnosis and treatment of attention deficit hyperactivity disorders. *Archives of Pediatrics and Adolescent Medicine*, *149*, 1211-1216.

Masse, L., Couture, C., and Anciaux, V. (2010). Knowledge and beliefs of professional workers in education, health and social services towards ADHD. *Sante Mentale ua Quebec*, *35* (1), 153-179.

MTA Cooperative Group (1999). A 14-month randomized clinical trial of treatment strategies for attention-deficit/hyperactivity disorder. *Archives of General Psychiatry*, *56*(12), 1073-86.

MTA Cooperative Group (2004). National Institute of Mental Health Multimodal Treatment Study of ADHD follow-up: 24-month outcomes of treatment strategies for attention-deficit/hyperactivity disorder. *Pediatrics*, *113* (4), 754-761.

National Institute for Health and Clinical Excellence (2008). *Attention deficit hyperactivity disorder: Diagnosis and management of ADHD in children, young people and adults*. Retrieved from http://www.nice.org.uk/CG72.

Pelham, W.E., Foster, M.E. and Robb, J.A. (2007). The economic impact of attention-deficit/hyperactivity disorder in children and adolescents. Journal of Psychiatric Psychology, 32,711-727.

Reeves, G., and Anthony, B. (2009). Multimodal treatments versus pharmacotherapy alone in children with psychiatric disorders: Implications of access, effectiveness, and contextual treatment. *Pediatric Drugs*, *11* (3), 165-169.

Roskin, G., Carsen, M.L., Rabiner, C.J., and Marell, S.K. (1988). Attitudes toward patients among different mental health professional groups. *Comprehensive Psychiatry*, *29*, 188-194.

Rowlandson, P.H. and Smith, C. (2009). An interagency service delivery model for autistic spectrum disorders and attention deficit hyperactivity disorder. Child: Care, Health and Development, 35,681-690.

Rushton, J.L., Fant, K.E., and Clark, S.J. (2004). Use of practice guidelines in the primary care of children with attention-deficit/hyperactivity disorder. *Pediatrics*, *114* (1), 23-28.

Shaw, K.A., Mitchell, G.K., Wagner, I.J. and Eastwood, H.L. (2002). Attitudes and practices of general practitioners in the diagnosis and management of attention-deficit/hyperactivity disorder.

Shaw, K. A., Wagner, I., Eastwood, H. and Mitchell, G. (2003). A qualitative study of Australian GPs' attitudes and practices in the diagnosis and management of attention-deficit/hyperactivity disorder (ADHD). *Family Practice*, *20* (2), 129-134.

Thapar, A., Holmes, J., Poulton, K., and Harrington, R. (1999). Genetic basis of attention deficit and hyperactivity. *British Journal of Psychiatry, 174*, 105-111.

Tyson, G.A., and Hubert, C. (2000). Australian adolescents' explanations of juvenile delinquency. *Australian Journal of Psychology, 52* (2), 119-124.

Weyandt, L.L., Fulton, K.M., Schepman, S.B., Verdi, G.R., and Wilson, K.G. (2009). Assessment of teacher and school psychologist knowledge of attention-deficit/hyperactivity disorder. *Psychology in Schools, 46* (10), 951-961.

Wolraich, M.L., Bard, D.E., Stein, M.T., Rushton, J.L., and O'Connor, K.G. (2010). Pediatrician's attitudes and practices on ADHD before and after the development of ADHD practice guidelines. *Journal of Attention Disorders, 13* (6), 563-572.

In: ADHD
Editors: R. Thompson and N. J. Miller
ISBN: 978-1-62417-107-9

Chapter 4

MOTOR COORDINATION DYSFUNCTION IN ADHD: NEW INSIGHTS FROM THE CLASSROOM TO GENETICS

Akio Nakai[*]
Associate Professor, Research Center for Child Mental Development, University of Fukui & Department of Child and Adolescent Psychological Medicine, University of Fukui Hospital, Fukui, Japan

ABSTRACT

Clinically, children with ADHD often have so-called "clumsiness", which means motor coordination dysfunction, and previous studies showed the high prevalence of comorbidity as 30~50%. This motor coordination problem is applicable to Developmental Coordination Disorder (DCD) in DSM-IV. Indeed, the results from our community-school based study, using the Japanese version of Developmental Coordination Disorder Questionnaire (DCDQ-J) and ADHD-Rating Scale (ADHD-RS-J), showed that all subscales and total scores of the DCDQ-J were significantly associated with the total and each subscales scores of ADHD-RS-J, which suggested that children with poor motor coordination more frequently showed inattention and hyperactivity.

[*] 23-3 Matsuoka-Shimoaizuki, Eiheiji-cho, Fukui, 910-1193, Japan; Phone: +81-776-61-3111, Fax: +81-776-61-8687; E-Mail : anakai@u-fukui.ac.jp

This frequent and specific comorbidity has led to new concepts or terms, such as DAMP (*Deficits in attention, motor control and perception*) syndrome (Gillberg, 2003), DCD-Plus (Gibbs, 2007), or different subtype of ADHD (Fliers, 2008). Gillberg, et al. reported a Swedish cohort study, which showed that 7.4% of all 7 year-old children had ADHD alone, 7.3% had DCD alone, and 6.6% had the DAMP syndrome, including 1.7% with a so-called 'severe' form. They also mentioned that the severe form of DAMP syndrome has also met criteria of the Autism spectrum disorder, including Asperger's syndrome. Lesson from our community-school based survey showed that, in Japan, 4.2% of children had ADHD alone, 3.8% had DCD alone, and 1.3% had the severe form of DAMP syndrome. Vice versa, 24% of children that had ADHD had DCD and 25% of children that had DCD had ADHD. The other way around, not all children with ADHD have motor coordination dysfunction. These facts might be one of the reasons that previous studies, such as SNPs or brain imaging, sometimes failed the constant and robust results, because of their heterogeneous subjects from these aspects.

While the recent brain imaging study revealed that lower rCBF of some brain lesions and different rCBF response to Methylphenidate were found in an ADHD comorbid DCD group compared to ADHD alone, and genome-wide association study suggested that *MAP2K5* and *CHD6*, and some SNPs might be involved in this combination.

New insights on the motor coordination dysfunction in ADHD from the classroom to genetics could lead to the new concept of disorder, and the new evidence-based diagnosis, medication or intervention.

1. Background

Clinically, children with attention-deficit hyperactivity disorder (ADHD) often have so-called "clumsiness", which means motor coordination dysfunction. This "clumsiness" affects various aspects in QOL of children with this impairment, not only in playing sports, gymnastics, and outdoor play, but also in daily life, such as eating, drinking, speaking, clothing, tying, drawing or writing, and playing musical instruments, etc. Previous studies showed the high prevalence of comorbidity or co-occurrence as 30~50% [1,2]. This motor coordination problem is applicable to Developmental Coordination Disorder (DCD) in DSM-IV (Diagnostic and statistical manual of mental disorders, 4th edition) [3], defined as "a marked impairment in the development of motor coordination, which interferes with daily living and studying."

DSM-IV [3] defines DCD according to the following four criteria:

A) Performance in daily activities that require motor coordination is substantially below that expected given the person's chronological age and measured intelligence. The disorder may be manifested by marked delays in motor milestones (e.g. walking, crawling, sitting), dropping things, 'clumsiness' and poor performance in sports or poor handwriting.
B) The disturbance described in criterion A significantly interferes with academic achievement or activities of daily living.
C) The disturbance is not due to a general medical condition (e.g. cerebral palsy, hemiplegia, or muscular dystrophy) and does not meet criteria for a pervasive developmental disorder.
D) If mental retardation is present, motor difficulties are in excess of those usually associated with mental retardation.

This frequent and specific comorbidity has led to some new terms, such as DAMP (*Deficits in attention, motor control and perception*) syndrome [4], DCD-Plus [5], or a different subtype of ADHD [6]. Besides, these comorbidities or co-occurrences of ADHD and DCD are revealed that the prognosis could be more severe than when each condition occurs separately [7-9].

In this chapter, I would like to introduce our community-school based survey of DAMP syndrome in Japan, and the recent studies in brain imaging and genetics. The lesson from classrooms and the recent advance in motor coordination dysfunction in ADHD could lead to new insights of this underestimated condition into new concepts or clinical entity.

2. Motor Coordination Dysfunction and ADHD: Lessons from the Classroom, in Japan

The purpose of this study was to describe the applicability of the Japanese version of Developmental Coordination Disorder Questionnaire (DCDQ-J) for use with a community-based population of children in Japan, and to investigate the relationships between motor coordination dysfunction and ADHD tendencies in Japanese children.

Kadesjö B and Gillberg C reported a Swedish cohort study which showed that 7.4% of all 7 year-old children had ADHD alone, 7.3% had DCD alone, and 6.6% had the DAMP syndrome, including 1.7% having a so-called 'severe' form [10] (Figure 1). They also mentioned that the severe form of DAMP syndrome has also met criteria of Autism spectrum disorder (ASD), including Asperger's syndrome.

The screening or assessment of motor dysfunction and ADHD in Japan could help us to identify the under-treatment of these problems in this country and to promote the new concept of the pathophysiology.

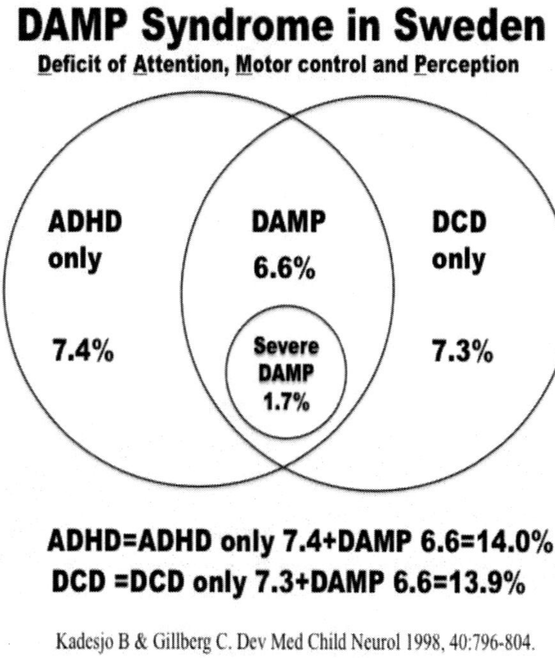

Figure 1. Estimated prevalence of ADHD, DCD and DAMP syndrome in Sweden.

2.1. Methods

2.1.1. Development of the Japanese version of the DCDQ (DCDQ-J)

The prevalence of DCD is about 6 to 10% world wide, and it is a common pediatric condition [3]. However, there is no international and standardized tool to facilitate the screening of DCD in Japan, which makes it difficult to evaluate the children's actual motor performance.

The Developmental Coordination Disorder Questionnaire (DCDQ) is a parent rating scale for screening pediatric DCD [11, 12]. DCDQ is a consisting of 15 items and was designed to screen for coordination disorders in children aged 5–15 years [11,12]. There are 3 subscales, namely, "control during movement (6 subitems)," "fine motor (4 subitems)," and "general coordination (5 subitems)." The descriptions of each item are scored as follows by a 5-point scale based on the comparison between the child and other (children): "Not at all like your child (1 point)," "A bit like your child (2 points)," "Moderately like your child (3 points)," "Quite a bit like your child (4 points)," and ""Extremely like your child (5 points)," with higher scores indicating better coordination. DCDQ has already translated into many languages, such as Hebrew, Chinese, Portuguese, and Danish.

Recently, we developed the Japanese version of the DCDQ (DCDQ-J) for the Japanese children [13]. A Japanese original questionnaire might be able to be developed, however, the World Health Organization (WHO) recommends the cross-cultural translation of existing instruments or questionnaires, because this process is efficient, faster and could facilitate the international collaboration, exchange of information and the cross-cultural comparisons. DCDQ-J has been developed in accordance with the International Guidelines [14]. We have conducted a preliminary investigation on both the reliability of DCDQ-J and the psychometric properties. The results indicated that the DCDQ-J could be a useful screening tool for DCD in Japan [13].

2.1.2. The Japanese version of the ADHD-Rating Scale (ADHD-RS-J)

We also employed the Japanese version of the ADHD-Rating Scale (ADHD-RS-J) developed by DuPaul, Power, Anastopoulos, & Reid [15, 16]. Based on the ADHD criteria of DSM-IV [3], this scale consists of 2 subscales to measure the 2 major characteristics of ADHD, namely, inattentiveness (9 items) and hyperactive-impulsiveness (9 items). Both the school and home forms of the ADHD-RS have been confirmed to have sufficient reliability and validity [15, 16, 17]. As in prior surveys, parents or rearers rated each item on a 4-point Likert scale ranging from "Not at all or rarely (0)" to "Sometimes (1)," "Often (2)," or "Very often (3)." Therefore, the higher a child's score, the more the ADHD tendency.

2.1.3. Participants

Our survey for so-called "DAMP syndrome in Japan" employed the DCDQ-J and ADHD-RS-J. Parents or guardians of all students in public nursery schools, elementary schools, and junior high schools in the participating city were invited to take part in this study. Nursery school students (middle class: 4- to 5-year-old students; senior class: 5- to 6-year-old students) and all elementary and junior high school students were included in this study. The questionnaire was sent to the parents or guardians via the teachers, with the sufficient instruction of DCDQ-J and ADHD-RS-J. The responses from the 6,330 respondents were analyzed. The majority (94%) of the respondents were mothers. Data from parents and guardians of children in special classrooms was excluded from the study. Table 1 shows the details of the children, as reported by the respondents.

Table 1. Details of grade and sex of participants

	Male	Female	Total
Nursery school (age band)			
Middle (4-5)	174	167	341
Senior (5-6)	154	176	330
Elementary school (age band)			
1 (6-7)	422	350	772
2 (7-8)	343	374	717
3 (8-9)	378	363	741
4 (9-10)	314	319	633
5 (10-11	328	352	680
6 (11-12)	310	292	602
Junior High school (age band)			
7 (12-13)	292	268	560
8 (13-14)	229	255	484
9 (14-15)	219	251	470
Total	3163	3167	6330

2.1.4. Procedure

The study was approved by the ethics committee. To request the cooperation of the target city, we provided the education committee of that city with an explanation of the purpose and method of our study, as well as an outline of our plan to protect the privacy of participants. We obtained consent from all of the preschools and elementary and junior high schools in the participating city and performed the survey using the described questionnaires.

2.2. Results

All subscales and total scores of the DCDQ-J were significantly associated with the total and each subscales scores of ADHD-RS-J, which suggested that children with poor motor coordination more frequently showed inattention and hyperactivity. Figure 2 shows the relationship between the total score of the Japanese version of DCDQ and ADHD-RS.

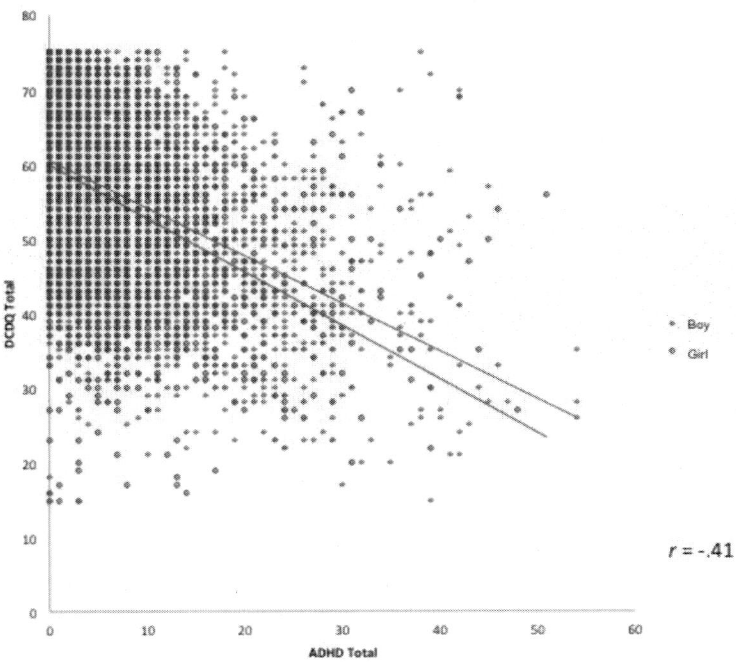

Figure 2. The relationship between total score of DCDQ-J and ADHD-RS-J.

Table 2. The Scores of the cut-off point of DAMP syndrome in Japan

	DCDQ-J				ADHD-RS-J			
	Male		Female		Male		Female	
	5%	15%	5%	15%	95%	85%	95%	85%
Nursery school								
Middle (4-5)	28.25	34.00	31.00	37.00	30.95	19.00	22.40	14.00
Senior (5-6)	30.70	41.00	32.45	40.00	25.75	20.25	21.75	12.25
Elementary school								
1 (6-7)	33.00	39.00	36.00	42.00	24.00	16.00	18.00	12.00
2 (7-8)	31.80	40.00	36.00	41.00	32.00	21.75	20.80	13.00
3 (8-9)	34.00	42.00	36.00	43.00	28.35	18.00	21.00	12.00
4 (9-10)	37.00	43.00	36.00	43.00	28.65	19.00	16.00	12.00
5 (10-11	36.15	43.00	37.00	44.00	28.75	17.00	17.00	11.00
6 (11-12)	33.40	41.00	38.00	44.90	24.00	16.00	16.00	11.00
Junior High school								
7 (12-13)	35.25	42.00	38.00	44.00	23.00	16.00	18.00	9.00
8 (13-14)	40.00	45.00	39.00	44.00	20.00	12.00	16.00	10.00
9 (14-15)	40.00	45.00	39.30	46.00	18.25	13.00	19.70	9.00
Total	34.00	41.00	36.00	43.00	26.00	17.00	18.00	12.00

With regard to the cut-off point of DCDQ-J, we adopted the 15th percentile and the 5th percentile, according to the statement of the Leeds Consensus 2006 [18]. In general, the 15th percentile of a screening questionnaire has been used to identify children "at risk" for motor problems. Those children "at risk" could have the difficulties with severe functional impairment, academic disruption, or co-existing developmental difficulties. To reach diagnostic criteria, the child must be below the 5th percentile, having significant functional impairment in activities of daily living or academic achievement. To keep consistency with DCDQ-J, we used the 85th percentile and the 95th percentile, respectively, for ADHD-RS-J. Table 2 showed the scores of each cut-off point for the screening of DAMP syndrome in Japan.

Table 3 and Figure 3 showed the prevalence of DAMP syndrome "at risk" in Japan, using the 15 percentile as the cut-off. For the screening, 5.8% of children had the tendency of DAMP syndrome in Japan, while 9.4% had ADHD alone and 9.9% had DCD alone. Concurrently, it could be said that 24% of ADHD had DCD, and 25% of DCD had ADHD. From the screening point of view in Japan, 15.2% of children have the tendency of ADHD (ADHD only 9.4% + DAMP 5.8%), and 15.7% of children DCD "at risk" (DCD only 9.9% + DAMP 5.8%), respectively.

Table 4 and Figure 4 showed the probable prevalence of DAMP syndrome in Japan, using the 5 percentile as the cut-off. The results, using more strict cut-off point, revealed that, in Japan, 4.2% of children had ADHD alone, 3.8% had DCD alone, and 1.3% had DAMP syndrome. Vice versa, 24% of children had ADHD had DCD and 25% of children that had DCD had ADHD. As well as the aspect using the 15 percentile, it is estimated, with the 5 percentile cut off, that in Japan, 5.4% of children could have ADHD (ADHD only 4.2% + DAMP 1.3%), and 5.1% of children could be suffering from DCD (DCD only 3.8 % + DAMP 1.3%), respectively.

2.3. Discussion

In this study, the DCDQ-J was related to the ADHD tendencies in the Japanese children. All subscales and total scores of the DCDQ-J were significantly associated with the ADHD-RS-J, which suggested that children with poor coordination more frequently showed inattention and hyperactivity.

Lesson from our community-school based survey revealed that, in Japan, 4.2% of children had ADHD alone, 3.8% had DCD alone, and 1.3% had DAMP syndrome. In addition, 24% of children with ADHD had DCD and 25% of children that had DCD had ADHD. The other way around, not all children with ADHD have motor coordination dysfunction.

This preliminary estimated prevalence of DAMP syndrome in Japan, using DCDQ-J and ADHD-RS-J, revealed to be similar to the reported prevalence in other countries.

Table 3. Estimated Prevalence of DAMP syndrome "at Risk" in Japan, using the cut-off with 15 percentile

		Total									
		DAMP		DCD only		ADHD only		Others		Total	
Nursery school											
	Middle (4-5)	21	(6.2)	33	(9.7)	34	(10.0)	253	(74.2)	341	(100)
	Senior (5-6)	16	(4.8)	36	(10.9)	29	(8.8)	249	(75.5)	330	(100)
Elementary school											
	1 (6-7)	53	(6.9)	67	(8.7)	76	(9.8)	576	(74.6)	772	(100)
	2 (7-8)	47	(6.6)	63	(8.8)	62	(8.6)	545	(76.0)	717	(100)
	3 (8-9)	38	(5.1)	86	(11.6)	80	(10.8)	537	(72.5)	741	(100)
	4 (9-10)	34	(5.4)	71	(11.2)	63	(10.0)	465	(73.5)	633	(100)
	5 (10-11	42	(6.2)	67	(9.9)	67	(9.9)	504	(74.1)	680	(100)
	6 (11-12)	36	(6.0)	54	(9.0)	56	(9.3)	456	(75.7)	602	(100)
Junior High school											
	7 (12-13)	31	(5.5)	59	(10.5)	57	(10.2)	413	(73.8)	560	(100)
	8 (13-14)	25	(5.2)	56	(11.6)	56	(11.6)	347	(71.7)	484	(100)
	9 (14-15)	24	(5.1)	53	(11.3)	55	(11.7)	338	(71.9)	470	(100)
	Total	370	(5.8)	627	(9.9)	595	(9.4)	4738	(74.8)	6330	(100)

		Total									
		DAMP		DCD only		ADHD only		Others		Total	
Nursery school											
	Middle (4-5)	8	(2.3)	11	(3.2)	7	(2.1)	315	(92.4)	341	(100)
	Senior (5-6)	1	(0.3)	14	(4.2)	14	(4.2)	301	(91.2)	330	(100)
Elementary school											
	1 (6-7)	6	(0.8)	37	(4.8)	36	(4.7)	693	(89.8)	772	(100)
	2 (7-8)	7	(1.0)	29	(4.0)	28	(3.9)	653	(91.1)	717	(100)
	3 (8-9)	10	(1.3)	28	(3.8)	26	(3.5)	677	(91.4)	741	(100)
	4 (9-10)	9	(1.4)	25	(3.9)	28	(4.4)	571	(90.2)	633	(100)
	5 (10-11	8	(1.2)	27	(4.0)	28	(4.1)	617	(90.7)	680	(100)
	6 (11-12)	13	(2.2)	17	(2.8)	20	(3.3)	552	(91.7)	602	(100)
Junior High school											
	7 (12-13)	7	(1.3)	22	(3.9)	23	(4.1)	508	(90.7)	560	(100)
	8 (13-14)	6	(1.2)	20	(4.1)	19	(3.9)	439	(90.7)	484	(100)
	9 (14-15)	8	(1.7)	19	(4.0)	14	(3.0)	429	(91.3)	470	(100)
	Total	83	(1.3)	239	(3.8)	267	(4.2)	5741	(90.7)	6330	(100)

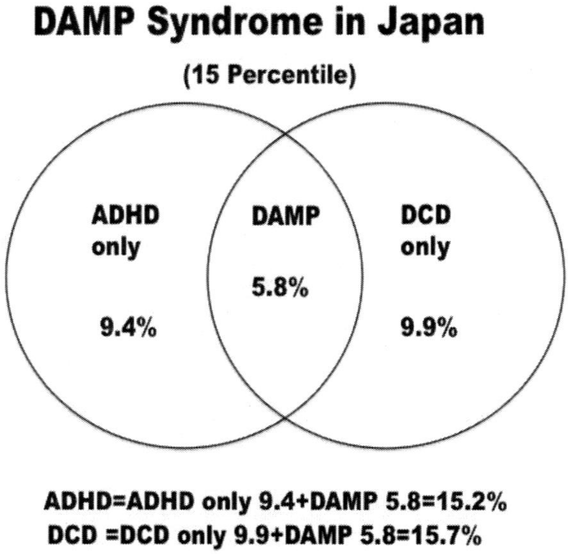

Figure 3. Estimated prevalence of DAMP syndrome "at risk" in Japan, using the 15 percentile as the cut-off.

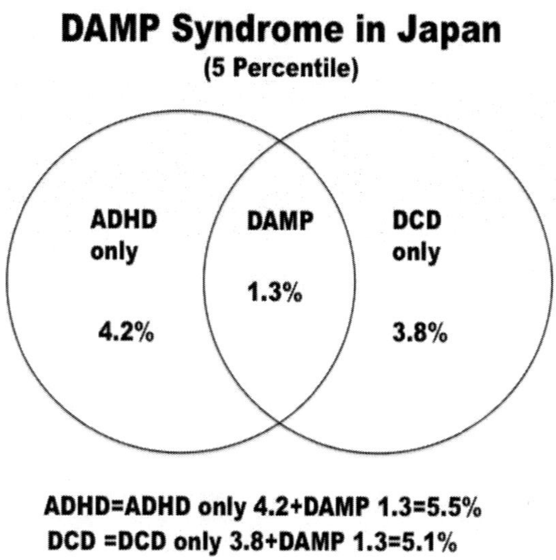

Figure 4. Estimated prevalence of DAMP syndrome in Japan, using the 5 percentile as the cut-off.

As mentioned above, a Swedish cohort study in 7 year-old children, reported by Kadesjo and Gillberg, showed that 7.4% had ADHD alone (moderate ADHD only; 5.4%, severe ADHD only; 2.0%), 7.3% had DCD alone (moderate or severe), and 6.6% had the DAMP syndrome, including 1.7% having a so-called 'severe' form [10]. In Canada, Dewey D, et al. reported that the children in both the 44.8% of DCD and 18.4% of DCD suspect groups have attention problems compared to children in the comparison group (3.5%) [19].

2.4. Limitations

Only the questionnaire survey was done in this study, which was not intended to provide a medical diagnosis of DCD and ADHD.

The European Academy for Childhood Disability (EACD) guideline [20] does not recommend the use of questionnaires for population-based screening for DCD, according to the report by Schoemaker MM. et al. with their low sensitivity in the general population [21].

Wilson BN, et al. confirmed, however, that the DCDQ is a valid clinical screening tool for DCD [12]. Correlations between DCDQ scores and Movement Assessment Battery for Children (r = .55) and Test of Visual-Motor Integration (r = .42) scores support concurrent validity [12]. In addition, EACD Recommendations also agrees that a questionnaire may be useful as a first step diagnostic tool. The DCDQ is so far the best-evaluated questionnaire [20]. It may be filled out by parents provided with sufficient instruction. In our study, 94% of the respondents of DCDQ-J and ADHD-RS-J were mothers.

2.5. Conclusions

Our lesson from the classroom emphasizes again that pediatricians and adolescent psychiatrists should pay more attention for movement impairments such as DCD, when assessing and treating ADHD, and new diagnostic categories in this aspect are necessary in the future.

3. The Possible Option for Interventions: Methylphenidate on Motor Functions in ADHD

Methylphenidate (MPH) is widely used in ADHD treatment. In contrast, the intervention or treatment of DCD is mainly the physical therapy or occupational therapy, including sensory integration, and the medication is rarely considered as the option.

However, it is reported that MPH could improve several aspects of motor functions in ADHD, such as fine motor function [22], handwriting [23], and postural stability and balance [24].

Bart O, et al. [25] studied the effects of MPH in children with comorbid DCD and ADHD, and found the significant improvement on the Movement Assessment Battery for Children (M-ABC) [26] scales for manual dexterity, ball skills, and dynamic balance tasks. In contrast, MPH was associated with only minor, not significant, improvement in static balance control. These results indicated that MPH might primarily affect the attention components of movement and motor planning. They stressed that clinically significant improvement by MPH was found in only 33% of the children. Flapper and Schoemaker reported that MPH significantly improved not only ADHD symptoms and motor functions, but also improved health-related quality of life (HRQOL), although additional motor therapy might still be needed in about half of the children with both ADHD and DCD [27].

The European Academy for Childhood Disability (EACD) recommended that MPH might be applied in children with DCD and comorbid ADHD to improve fine motor symptoms. They need additional treatment and support to overcome specific functional problems for handwriting and drawing [20].

These studies, except for Flapper and Schoemaker [27], included the children already being treated with MPH, so that the results were sometimes variable. However, some recent studies in drug-naive children have confirmed that MPH have effects not only in fine motor skills or hand writing, but also many aspects of motor functions. Stray LL, et al. [28] reported that a single dose of 10 mg MPH markedly improved motor functions of drug-naive children with ADHD in neuro-motor inhibition, or tonus in the gross movement muscles, involved in maintaining the alignment and balance of the body. A cohort study of 49 drug-naive children with ADHD was conducted for the long-term effects of MPH [29]. Children were evaluated, using the Movement Assessment Battery for Children (M-ABC) [26] and the developmental test of visual motor integration at diagnosis and after MPH treatment. They showed that three months of treatment with MPH improves motor skills in around 20% of the children. Nevertheless, motor impairment persisted in more than half of the children.

As described in EACD guideline [20], further studies should be done to measure the effect of MPH on a larger group of not only children with DCD and ADHD, but also children with DCD without ADHD. A randomized controlled trial with a follow-up over a longer period of time should be needed.

MPH might have the effects not only on ADHD symptoms, but also on the motor coordination dysfunctions, via cortico-striatal dopaminergic system. On the other side, atomoxetine is a selective norepinephrine reuptake inhibitor. Noradrenergic neurons project form the locus ceruleus to the whole brain system, including the cerebellum, in which there is no dopaminergic innervation. Although there are little studies on the effects of atomoxetine on motor functions of ADHD, it is suspected that atomoxetine might be effective to motor impairments in ADHD, through the different mechanism from MPH.

4. Brain Imaging Studies on ADHD with DCD

It is suspected the comorbidity or co-occurrence of ADHD and DCD might be a new clinical entity, although the neurobiological pathophysiology of these motor dysfunctions of ADHD remains unclear. The objective and quantitative biological markers for evidence-based diagnosis and interventions to reduce the risk for poor outcomes need to be developed. Brain imaging studies, such as structural or functional imaging, could help to understand these issues.

Motor skills are related to the many brain lesions, including cerebrum, cerebellum and motor neuron to neuromuscular junction and muscle sensors and cells. And the motor coordination consists of perceptual, feedback and learning processes, motor preparation and movement execution processes. These processes rely on the visual, memory, attention, the balance, the kinaesthetic and the motor effector system.

In the aspect of ADHD, meta-analysis of structural MRI studies detected basal ganglia regions like the right globus pallidus, the right putamen, and the caudate are affected in children with ADHD [30]. In a recent review of DCD, the brain imaging studies revealed that the broad network of regions was associated with motor learning, including bilateral inferior parietal lobules, right dorsolateral prefrontal cortex, and the cerebellum [31].

Thus, there are several common brain lesions involved both in ADHD and DCD while a few studies have been reported studying the comorbidity or co-occurrence of ADHD and DCD conditions. Recently, however, two brain imaging studies were published; one using technetium-99m ethyl cysteinate dimmer (99mTc-ECD) single photon emission computed tomography (SPECT) [32], and another using the technique of the transcranial magnetic stimulation (TMS)–evoked short interval cortical inhibition (SICI) in motor cortex [33].

The former study was done in drug-naive adolescents with ADHD with or without DCD [32]. The baseline and changes of regional cerebral blood flow (rCBF) after MPH challenge between two groups were compared. In the baseline evaluation, rCBF were lower in the bilateral frontal lobe, inferior parental lobe, and increased rCBF of right posterior cingulate gyrus, anterior lobe of cerebellum were found in ADHD with DCD group, compared to ADHD alone. After 10 mg of MPH, rCBF decreased in the right occipital, inferior temporal lobe in ADHD with DCD group, while the ADHD-alone group showed increments of rCBF in the bilateral occipital lobe.

The latter study was done with 49 children with ADHD and 49 control children [33]. Motor skills were evaluated with the Physical and Neurological Examination for Subtle Signs (PANESS) and the Motor Assessment Battery for Children- 2nd version (M-ABC2) [34]. SICI were obtained using TMS in the left motor cortex. Reduced TMS-evoked SICI correlates with ADHD diagnosis and symptom severity and also reflects motor skills. It is reported that SICI is related with γ-aminobutyric acid (GABA) A-mediated inhibition, so that the further studies are needed to evaluate the interactions of GABA and dopamine in motor dysfunction in ADHD.

5. Genetic Studies on ADHD with DCD

ADHD is a heterogeneous condition. It is suggested, however, that ADHD is a heritable disorder from a large number of family and twin studies. Although the mechanism of the genetics of ADHD remain unclear, the polygenic transmission model is suspected [35]. Two approaches have been available currently: one is the hypothesis-driven candidate gene association study, and the other is the hypothesis-free genome-wide linkage analysis. At this time, the results of both approaches have failed to identify the major genes for ADHD [36].

A recent meta-analytic review showed that significant heterogeneity was observed for the associations between ADHD and *DAT1, DRD4. DRD5, DBH, ADRA2A, 5HTT, TPH2, MAOA,* and *SNAP25,* and individual gene variants have only shown small effects, rarely reaching an odds ratio of around 1.3 [37]. Meta-analysis of the linkage studies only confirmed one locus, on chromosome 16 [38].

However, the recent genome-wide association study, focused on this combination of ADHD and DCD, revealed the possible relationships between the phenotype and some genes, such as *MAP2K5* and *CHD6*. Further characterization of these findings using DCDQ subscales found nominal association for some single nucleotide polymorphism (SNP), such as the SNP rs11002745, and SNP rs2839083 [39].

The *MAP2K5*, a member of the mitogen-activated protein kinase family, is suggested to be involved in neuroprotection of dopaminergic neurons. It is known that *MAP2K5* has been associated with restless legs syndrome (RLS). Clinically, up to 44% of subjects with ADHD have RLS or RLS symptoms, and up to 26% of RLS patients have ADHD, vice versa [40], and it is also reported that RLS and ADHD share common risk genes [41]. Deletion of the *CHD6* exon 12 affects motor coordination in a mouse model [42]. The SNP rs11002745 showed association with gross motor problems, and the SNP rs2839083 was associated with fine motor problems and control during movement. SNP rs2839083 is located 18.7 kb downstream of the *COL6A1* gene on chromosome 21 [39]. Mutations in *COL6A1* gene are known to cause motor problems in collagen-type VI-related disorders [43].

Conclusions

The lesson of our school-based survey in Japan revealed that children with ADHD tendency have motor coordination dysfunction, as well. The estimated prevalence of this unique comorbidity, so-called "DAMP syndrome" is the same as the results of the previous studies. It is reported that these comorbidities or co-occurrences of ADHD and DCD could lead tomore severe prognosis than when each condition occurs separately. We, clinicians should pay more attention to motor impairments in ADHD, when diagnosing and treating children. MPH have the effects not only on the core symptoms of ADHD, but also on the several aspects of motor coordination, such as gross motor, fine motor or handwriting, balance, and muscle tones. On the other hand, however, not all children with ADHD have motor coordination dysfunction. The recent brain imaging and genetic studies showed the possibilities of the new clinical entity of this comorbidity.

New insights on the motor coordination dysfunction in ADHD from the classroom to genetics could lead to the new concept of disorder, and the evidence-based diagnosis, medication or intervention.

Acknowledgments

The author has no conflict of interests to declare. This study was supported, in part, by a Research Grant from the Ministry of Health, Labour and Welfare, Japan, and Grant-in-Aid for Scientific Research from the Japan Society for the Promotion of Science. The author is grateful to the children and parents who participated. The author also thanks Dr. Masafumi Ohnishi (University of Fukui, Japan), for assistance of this study, and Dr. Brenda N. Wilson (Alberta Health Services and University of Calgary, Canada) for the approval for use of the DCDQ. ADHD-RS Japanese version was used by the courtesy and the permission of Prof. Yasuo Tanaka, Hokkaido University, Japan. The author thanks Kate Tomanelli, Nova Science Publishers, Inc. for English-language editing.

References

[1] Polatajko, H.J., Cantin, N. (2005). Developmental coordination disorder (dyspraxia): an overview of the state of the art. *Seminars in Pediatric Neurology*. 12, 250–258.

[2] Fliers, E., Rommelse, N., Vermeulen, S.H., Altink, M., Buschgens, C.J., Faraone, S.V., Sergeant, J.A., Franke, B., Buitelaar, J.K. (2008). Motor coordination problems in children and adolescents with ADHD rated by parents and teachers: effects of age and gender. *Journal of Neural Transmission*. 115, 211-20.

[3] American Psychological Association. (2000). Diagnostic and statistical manual of mental disorders: DSM-IV-TR. (4th ed.). Washington, DC.

[4] Gillberg, C. (2003). Deficits in attention, motor control, and perception: a brief review. *Archives of Disease in Childhood*. 88:904-910.

[5] Gibbs, J., Appleton, J., Appleton, R. (2007). Dyspraxia or developmental coordination disorder? Unravelling the enigma. *Archives of Disease in Childhood. 92*, 534-539.

[6] Fliers, E., Vermeulen, S., Rijsdijk, F. (2009). ADHD and poor motor performance from a family genetic perspective. *Journal of the American Academy of Child & Adolescent Psychiatry*. 48, 25–34.

[7] Gillberg, C. (1992). Deficits in attention, motor control and perception, and other syndromes attributed to minimal brain dysfunction. In J. Aicardi (Ed.), Diseases of the nervous system in children. Clinics in developmental medicine. London: MacKeith.

[8] Pitcher, T., Piek, J., Hay, D. (2003). Fine and gross motor ability in males with ADHD. *Developmental Medicine and Child Neurology*, 45, 525–535.

[9] Visser, J. (2003). Developmental coordination disorder: A review of research on subtypes and comorbidities. *Human Movement Science*. 22, 479–493.

[10] Kadesjö, B., Gillberg, C. (1998). Attention deficits and clumsiness in Swedish 7-year-old children. *Developmental Medicine and Child Neurology*. 40, 796-804.

[11] Wilson, B.N., Kaplan, B.J., Crawford, S.G., Campbell, A., Dewey, D. (2000). Reliability and validity of a parent questionnaire on childhood motor skills, *American Journal of Occupational Therapy*. 54, 484-493.

[12] Wilson, B.N., Crawford, S.G., Green, D., Roberts, G., Aylott, A., Kaplan, B.J. (2009). Psychometric properties of the revised Developmental Coordination Disorder Questionnaire, *Physical & Occupational Therapy in Pediatrics*. 29, 182-202.

[13] Nakai, A., Miyachi, T., Okada, R., Tani, I., Nakajima, S., Onishi, M., Fujita, C., Tsujii, M. (2011). Evaluation of the Japanese version of the Developmental Coordination Disorder Questionnaire as a screening tool for clumsiness of Japanese children. *Research in Developmental Disabilities*. 32, 1615-22.

[14] Beaton, D., Bombardier, C., Guillemin, F., Feraz, M.B. (2000). Guidelines for process of cross-cultural adaptation of self-report measures. *Spine*. 25, 3186–3191.

[15] DuPaul, G.J., Power, T.J., Anastopoulos, A., Reid, R. (1998). ADHD Rating Scale-IV: Checklists, norms, and clinical interpretation, Guilford Press, New York, USA.

[16] DuPaul, G.J., Power, T.J., McGoey, K.E., Ikeda, M.J., Anastopoulos, A.D. (1998). Reliability and validity of parent and teacher ratings of attention deficit hyperactivity disorder symptoms. *Journal of Psychoeducational Assessment*. 16, 55–68.

[17] DuPaul, G.J., Power, T.J., Anastopoulos, A., Reid, R. (2008). ADHD Rating Scale-IV: Checklists, norms, and clinical interpretation (Ichikawa, H., Tanaka, Y. Trans.), Akashi-shoten, Tokyo, Japan (Original work published 1998) (in Japanese).

[18] LEEDS CONSENSUS STATEMENT (2006). ESRC Seminar Series Developmental Coordination Disorder LEEDS 2004-2005. http://www.dcd-uk.org/

[19] Dewey, D., Kaplan, B.J., Crawford, S.G., Wilson, B.N. (2002). Developmental coordination disorder: associated problems in attention, learning, and psychosocial adjustment. *Human Movement Science*. 21, 905-18.

[20] Blank, R., Smits-Engelsman, B., Polatajko, H., Wilson, P. European Academy for Childhood Disability. (2012). European Academy for Childhood Disability (EACD): Recommendations on the definition, diagnosis and intervention of developmental coordination disorder (long version). *Developmental Medicine and Child Neurology*. 54, 54-93.

[21] Schoemaker, M.M., Flapper, B., Verheij, N.P., Wilson, B.N., Reinders-Messelink, H.A., de Kloet, A. (2006). Evaluation of the Developmental Coordination Disorder Questionnaire as a screening instrument. *Developmental Medicine and Child Neurology*. 48, 668-73.

[22] Flapper, B.C., Houwen, S., Schoemaker, M.M. (2006). Fine motor skills and effects of methylphenidate in children with attention deficit hyperactivity disorder and developmental coordination disorder. *Developmental Medicine and Child Neurology*. 48, 165–169.

[23] Lange, K.W., Tucha, L., Walitza, S., Gerlach, M., Linder, M., Tucha, O. (2007). Interaction of attention and graphomotor functions in children with attention deficit hyperactivity disorder. *Journal of Neural Transmission*. 72, 249–259.

[24] Jacobi-Polishook, T., Shorer, Z., Melzer, I. (2009). The effect of methylphenidate on postural stability under single and dual task conditions in children with attention deficit hyperactivity disorder—A double blind randomized control trial. *Journal of the Neurological Sciences*. 280, 15–21.

[25] Bart, O., Podoly, T., Bar-Haim, Y. (2010). A preliminary study on the effect of methylphenidate on motorperformance in children with comorbid DCD and ADHD. *Research in Developmental Disabilities*. 31,1443–1447.

[26] Henderson, S.E., Sugden, D.A. (1992). Movement Assessment Battery for Children: manual. The Psychological Corporation Ltd. London, UK.

[27] Flapper, B.C., Schoemaker, M.M. (2008). Effects of methylphenidate on quality of life in children with both developmental coordination disorder and ADHD. *Developmental Medicine and Child Neurology*. 50, 294-9.

[28] Stray, L.L., Stray, T., Iversen, S., Ruud, A., Ellertsen, B. (2009). Methylphenidate improves motor functions in children diagnosed with Hyperkinetic Disorder. *Behavioral and Brain Functions*. 5:21 doi:10.1186/1744-9081-5-21

[29] Brossard-Racine, M., Shevell, M., Snider, L., Ageranioti Be´ langer, S., Majnemer, A. (2012). Motor skills of children newly diagnosed with attention deficit hyperactivity disorder prior to and following treatment with stimulant medication. *Research in Developmental Disabilities*. 33, 2080–2087.

[30] Frodl, T., Skokauskas, N. (2012). Meta-analysis of structural MRI studies in children and adults with attention deficit hyperactivity disorder indicates treatment effects. *Acta Psychiatrica Scandinavica*. 125, 114-26.

[31] Zwicker, J.G., Missiuna, C., Harris, S.R., Boyd, L.A. (2012). Developmental coordination disorder: A review and update. *European Journal of Pediatric Neurology*. http://dx.doi.org/10.1016/ j.ejpn.2012.05.005,

[32] Yeh, C.B., Huang, W.S., Lo, M.C., Chang, C.J., Ma, K.H., Shyu, J.F. (2012). The rCBF brain mapping in adolescent ADHD comorbid developmental coordination disorder and its changes after MPH challenging. *European Journal of Pediatric Neurology*. [Epub ahead of print]

[33] Gilbert, D.L., Isaacs, K.M., Augusta, M., MacNeil, L.K., Mostofsky, S.H. (2011). TMS Motor cortex inhibition; A marker of ADHD behavior and motor development in children. *Neurology*. 76, 615–621.

[34] Henderson, S.E., Sugden, D.A., Barnett, A.L. (2007). Movement Assessment Battery for Children – second edition (Movement ABC-2); examiner's manual. Harcourt Assessment, London, UK.

[35] Faraone, S.V., Perlis, R.H., Doyle, A.E., Smoller, J.W., Goralnick, J.J., Holmgren, M.A., Sklar, P. (2005). Molecular genetics of attention deficit hyperactivity disorder. *Biological Psychiatry*. 57:1313–1323

[36] Gizer, I.R., Ficks, C., Waldman, I.D. (2009). Candidate gene studies of ADHD: a meta-analytic review. *Human Genetics*. 126, 51–90.

[37] Zhou, K., Dempfle, A., Arcos-Burgos, M., Bakker, S.C., Banaschewski, T., Biederman, J., Buitelaar, J., Castellanos, F.X., Doyle, A., Ebstein, R.P., Ekholm, J., Forabosco, P., Franke, B., Freitag, C., Friedel, S., Gill, M., Hebebrand, J., Hinney, A., Jacob, C., Lesch, K.P., Loo, S.K., Lopera, F., McCracken, J.T., McGough, J.J., Meyer, J., Mick, E., Miranda, A., Muenke, M., Mulas, F., Nelson, S.F., Nguyen, T.T., Oades, R.D., Ogdie, M.N., Palacio, J.D., Pineda, D., Reif, A., Renner, T.J., Roeyers, H., Romanos, M., Rothenberger, A., Schafer, H., Sergeant, J., Sinke, R.J., Smalley, S.L., Sonuga-Barke, E., Steinhausen, H.C., van der Meulen, E., Walitza, S., Warnke, A., Lewis, C.M., Faraone, S.V., Asherson, P. (2008). Meta-analysis of genome-wide linkage scans of attention deficit hyperactivity disorder. *American Journal of Medical Genetics Part B: Neuropsychiatric Genetics*. 147B, 1392–1398.

[38] Franke, B., Neale, B.M., Faraone, S.V. (2009). Genome-wide association studies in ADHD. *Human Genetics*. 126, 13-50.

[39] Fliers, E.A., Vasquez, A.A., Poelmans, G., Rommelse, N., Altink, M., Buschgens, C., Asherson, P., Banaschewski, T., Ebstein, R., Gill, M., Miranda, A., Mulas, F., Oades, R.D., Roeyers, H., Rothenberger, A., Sergeant, J., Sonuga-Barke, E., Steinhausen, H.C., Faraone, S.V., Buitelaar, J.K., Franke, B. (2012). Genome-wide association study of motor coordination problems in ADHD identifies genes for brain and muscle function. *World Journal of Biological Psychiatry*. 13, 211-22.

[40] Cortese, S., Konofal, E., Lecendreux, M., Arnulf, I., Mouren, M.C., Darra, F., Dalla Bernardina, B. (2005). Restless legs syndrome and attention deficit hyperactivity disorder: a review of the literature. *Sleep*. 28, 1007-13.

[41] Schimmelmann, B.G., Friedel, S., Nguyen, T.T., Sauer, S., Ganz Vogel, C.I., Konrad, K., Wilhelm, C., Sinzig, J., Renner, T.J., Romanos, M., Palmason, H., Dempfle, A., Walitza, S., Freitag, C., Meyer, J., Linder, M., Schäfer, H., Warnke, A., Lesch, K.P., Herpertz-Dahlman, B., Hinney, A., Hebebrand, J. (2009). Exploring the genetic link between RLS and ADHD. *Journal of Psychiatric Research*. 43, 941-5.

[42] Lathrop, M.J., Chakrabarti, L., Eng, J., Rhodes, C.H., Lutz, T., Nieto, A., Liggitt, H.D., Warner, S., Fields, J., Stöger, R., Fiering, S. (2010). Deletion of the Chd6 exon 12 affects motor coordination. *Mammalian Genome*. 21, 130-142.

[43] Lampe, A.K., Flanigan, K.M., Bushby, K.M. (2004). Collagen Type VI-Related Disorders. Editors In: Pagon, R.A., Bird, T.D., Dolan, C.R., Stephens, K., Adam, M.P., editors. GeneReviews™ [Internet]. Seattle (WA): University of Washington, Seattle, USA.

In: ADHD
Editors: R. Thompson and N. J. Miller
ISBN: 978-1-62417-107-9

Chapter 5

Importance of Nutrition Optimization in Multimodal Treatment in Children with Attention-Deficit Hyperactivity Disorder

Teodoro Durá-Travé*,
María Eugenia Yoldi-Petri
and Fidel Gallinas-Victoriano
Neurology Pediatric Unit, Navarra Hospital Complex,
Pamplona, Spain

Abstract

Background. Multimodal treatment of attention-deficit hyperactivity disorder (ADHD) combines psychosocial intervention with drug therapy, which, generally, involves a long-term administration of stimulant drugs. Methylphenidate has consistent efficacy with respect to the cardinal symptoms of ADHD and its comorbidity, even though there is some controversy concerning the potential negative influence this drug has on the growth in these patients. This study presents an evolutionary analysis of anthropometric variables in a group of patients diagnosed with ADHD

* Address correspondence: Navarra Hospital Complex, Neurology Pediatric Unit, T. Durá-Travé, Avenue Irunlarrea, 4. CP:31008 Pamplona, Spain, E-mail: tduratra@cfnavarra.es, Fax: 848 42 99 24, Tel. 848 42 25 63

in order to determine the repercussion of drug therapy with osmotic release oral system methylphenidate (OROS-methylphenidate) on the weight and height curve of these patients. The consequences of this nutrition optimization are analyzed.

Patients and methods. Clinical records of 187 patients with ADHD under treatment with OROS-methylphenidate during 30 months (first stage) were reviewed. Weight, height and body mass index values at diagnosis (basal) and after 6, 12, 18, 24 and 30 months of treatment were registered. Subsequently, patients followed a nutritional intervention and weight, height and body mass index were prospectively recorded after 36, 42 and 48 months of follow up (second stage).

Results. Mean age at diagnosis was 8.14 ± 1.6 years. Mean dose of OROS-methylphenidate was gradually increased, from 0.89 ± 0.21 mg/kg/day after 6 months of treatment to 1.05 ± 0.2 mg/kg/day after 30 months (first stage), and 1.31± 0.2 mg/kg/day after 48 months of follow up (second stage). Mean weight at diagnosis was lower than expected mean weight for age in 0.697 kg (weight deficit). This difference increased to 4.274 kg (1.43 kg/year) after 30 months of treatment (first stage), subsequently decreased and was 1.588 kg (0.22 kg/year) after 48 months of treatment (second stage). In the same way, mean height values for these patients at diagnosis were lower than expected mean height values for age in 0.42 cm (height deficit). This difference increased to 2.69 cm (0.91 cm/year) after 30 months of treatment (first stage), subsequently decreased and was 0.83 (0.1 cm/year) after 48 months of follow up (second stage).

Conclusions. Daily treatment with OROS-methylphenidate in patients diagnosed with ADHD has a negative impact in anthropometric variables (weight and height), but the application of nutrition optimization strategies allows recovering weight and height deficit. Nutrition education programs should join multimodal treatments in these patients in order to lessen nutritional problems and the consequences that could be derived from treatment with OROS-methylphenidate.

INTRODUCTION

Attention deficit hyperactivity disorder (ADHD) is a heterogeneous behavioral disorder with an estimated prevalence of 5-9% within the pediatric population [1-3]. It is characterized by inattention, hyperactivity and impulsivity and associated with social, educational and/or psychological deterioration [4-8]. In addition, a variable percentage of patients show comorbid disorders that complicate diagnosis and treatment efficacy [5, 9].

Multimodal treatment of ADHD requires psychosocial intervention as well as drug therapy, which, generally, implies a long-term administration of stimulant drugs [5, 9-11] as first choice treatment. In Spain, methylphenidate (MPH), in its different pharmacokinetic formulations (immediate and sustained release), is the only available stimulant drug. Osmotic-controlled release oral delivery system methylphenidate (OROS-MPH) tablets provide a quick plasmatic concentration (in two or three hours), followed by a prolonged and ascending release with a maximum plasmatic concentration in 6-8 hours and a duration of therapeutic effect of 12 hours; in other words, it guarantees a more constant therapeutic response avoiding the peaks and subsequent falls in plasmatic concentrations which are usual in immediate release formulation. Methylphenidate works as a catecholamine reuptake inhibitor, and so increases catecholamine levels (dopamine and norepinephrine) into the synaptic cleft. Methylphenidate has consistent efficacy with regards to the cardinal symptoms of ADHD and its comorbidity [11-15]. There is some controversy regarding the potential negative influence this drug has on anthropometric variables (weight and height) in these patients [16-25], whose mechanism of action was related with increased extra synaptic levels of dopamine in hypothalamus and striatum[26, 27]. The estimated high prevalence of patients diagnosed with ADHD subject to treatment with methylphenidate, together with a common concern with a potential negative effect of methylphenidate on growth curve, accounts for the evolutionary analysis of the anthropometric variables in a group of patients with ADHD under treatment with sustained-release methylphenidate. This study presents an evolutionary analysis of anthropometric variables in a group of patients diagnosed with ADHD with the aim of determining the repercussion of drug therapy with osmotic release oral system methylphenidate (OROS-MPH) during 4 years on the weight and height curve of these patients. The importance of nutritional intervention is evaluated.

Material and Methods

The study consists of two different stages: a first stage as a retrospective evaluation (30 months long) and, after nutrition intervention, a second stage as a prospective follow up (18 months long).

Patients

In the first stage, we made a random retrospective revision of clinical records from 201 patients diagnosed with ADHD under continuous treatment with OROS-MPH. The interval included the time of diagnosis to 30 months later. They were required to have been clinically evaluated in our department within the period June-December, 2008. The application of the Diagnostic and Statistical Manual of Mental Disorders (DSM IV-R) [28] criteria allowed diagnosis and classification. Patients were separated in two clinical subtypes: those who mainly manifest attention deficit or *inattentive subtype* and those with attention deficit, hyperactivity and impulsivity or *combined subtype*.

All those patients who ceased treatment during school holidays or summer periods were excluded. The resulting study sample was 187 patients. Diagnostic procedure included blood tests (complete blood count, serum biochemistry profile including liver function tests, thyroid hormone tests, etc.) in 72 patients (38.5%), genetic studies in 7 patients (3.7%), neurophysiological tests in 53 patients (28.3%) and neuroimaging procedures in 65 patients (34.8%). After the collection of the results of this first stage, we proceeded to design a nutrition intervention.

We contacted every primary health care pediatrician responsible for these patients and summoned them to an up-to-date meeting, where most of them met up. The Scientific program included the presentation of the results of the first stage under the title "*Nutritional features in Attention Deficit Hyperactivity Disorder*". In this meeting, we remarked the importance of the systematic record of anthropometric variables (weight, height and body mass index) and their comparison with appropriate reference patterns (growth charts and curves). We asked explicitly for collaboration in the nutrition optimization of these patients through the application of nutrition strategies, such as increasing breakfast or dinner calorie intake, offering favorite foods for lunch and/or adding calorie supplements. In the second stage, these 187 patients were periodically evaluated during 18 months until the fulfillment of 48 months of treatment.

Nutrition Study

Nutrition study was similar in both stages. Different variables were collected from every clinical record: sex, age, clinical subtype, OROS-MPH dose (mg/kg/day), weight and height at diagnosis and at follow-up examinations after 6, 12, 18, 24, 30 months (first stage), and after 36, 42 and 48 months (second stage). Weight and height measurements were recorded with patients wearing only underwear and no shoes. An Año-Sayol® scale was used for weight measurement, with a measuring range of 0 to 120 kg and a precision of 100 g. Height was measured on a rigid wall mounted stadiometer with a range 60 to 210 cm, and a precision of 0.1 cm.

Weight z-score, height z-score and body mass index (BMI) z-score, as well as their expected (z-score equals zero) weight and height for age and sex were recorded in every patient after the referred follow-up examinations. The SEINAPTRACKER (Medicalsoft Intercath, S.L. University of Barcelona, 2007-2008) computer program was used to perform these calculations. The growth charts and data tables of "Centro Andrea Prader" (Zaragoza, 2002) were used as standard references. This research protocol has been approved by the Ethics Committee of the "Navarra Hospital Complex". Results are showed as means with the corresponding confidence intervals (95% CI) or standard deviations (SD). The computer program SPSS 17.0 for Windows (Chicago, Illinois, USA) was used to perform the statistical analysis (Student's test, $\chi 2$ test and Pearson coefficient correlation).

Results

The sample consisted of 129 males (69%) and 58 females (31%), with a male/female ratio of 2.2. The combined subtype (n=158) represented 84.5% of the cases and the inattentive subtype (n=29) was 15.5%. The proportion of combined subtype was significantly higher ($p<0.001$) in males (89.9%) than in females (72.4%) (Table 1). Mean age at diagnosis was 8.14±1.6 years. Diagnosis was achieved in school age (6-10 years) in 84.5% of patients, preschool age (<6 years) in 10.5% of patients and adolescence (>10 years) in 5% of patients (figure 1).

We did not find any significant differences in age at diagnosis regarding sex (males: 8.08±1.64 years, females: 8.29±1.52 years) and clinical subtype (combined: 8.15±1.64 years, inattentive: 8.08 ±1.44 years). Anthropometric variables' recording was made after a period of 6.3±1.5, 12.1±1.5, 17.8±1.4, 23.7±1.5 and 29.9±1.2 months of treatment. The results of the blood, genetic, neurophysiologic and neuroimaging studies were considered normal, except for the finding of agenesis of the corpus callosum in one patient.

Table 2 shows mean values of age, as well as OROS-MPH dose (mg/kg/day) and BMI (z-scores) of these patients in every evolutionary follow up. The daily mean dose of OROS-MPH (mg/kg/d) was gradually increased during the follow up period. From a mean dose of 0.89±0.21 after six months, it reached 1.31±0.2 after 48 months of follow up ($p<0.05$).

Table 1. Distribution of clinical subtypes according to sex

Clinical subtype	Combined	Inattentive	Total
Males	118	11	129
Females	42	16	58
Total	160	27	187

X^2=11.76 ($p<.001$).

Table 2. Mean values for age, OROS-MPH dose and BMI in patients along treatment

Evolution (n)	Age (years) X (SD)	Dose (mg/kg/d) X (SD)	BMI (Z-score) X (SD
Basal (n=187)	8.14 (1.60)	---	-0.14 (0.97
6 months (n=152)	8.66 (1.65)	0.89 (0.21)	-0.50 (0.82)*
12 months (n=158)	9.18 (1.44)	0.90 (0.24)	-0.47 (0.77)*
18 months (n=151)	9.69 (1.68)	0.95 (0.25)	-0.56 (0.82)*
24 months (n=164)	10.01 (1.55)	1.02 (0.24)*	-0.42 (0.94)*
30 months (n=149)	10.69 (1.64)	1.05 (0.23)*	-0.49 (0.98)*
36 months (n=165)	11.13 (1.44)	1.24 (0.18)*	-0.45 (0.93)*
42 months (n=148)	11.53 (1.51)	1.25 (0.20)*	-0.28 (0.97)
48 months (n=160)	12.09 (1.50)	1.31 (0.20)*	-0.20 (0.99)

*$p<0.05$ with respect to basal value.

Mean BMI values (z-score) maintained significantly lower ($p<0.05$) than basal value until 36 months of follow-up, and recovered subsequently. Table 3 displays mean values of weight and height, and the differences between expected weight and height for age (when z-score was 0) and registered weight and height in every follow-up control (weight deficit and height deficit, respectively). In absolute terms, mean values of weight and height increased progressively.

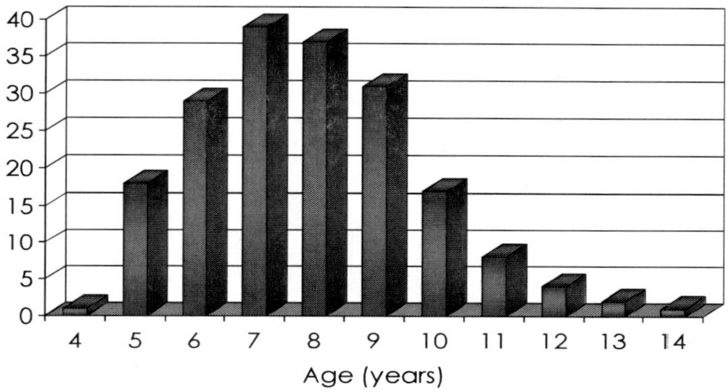

Figure 1. Distribution of age at diagnosis.

Table 3. Mean values for registered weight and height and weight and height deficit along treatment

Time (months)	Height X (95% CI)	Weight X (95% CI)	Weight deficit X (95% CI)	Height deficit X (95% CI)
Basal (n=187)	129.30 (127.97-130.63)	27.61 (26.88-28.34)	0,697 (0.35-1.04)	0.42 (0.1-0.83)
6 (n=152)	132.05 (130.68-133.42)	28.03 (27.23-28.83)	2.218* (1.55-2.87)	0.42 (0.01-0.08)
12 (n=158)	133.37 (132.23-134.51)	29.32 (28.40-30.24)	2.864* (2.37-3.35)	1.05 (0.65-1.45)
18 (n=151)	135.44 (133.91-136.97)	30.16 (29.15-31.17)	3.724* (3.02-4.42)	1.73 (0.98-2.46)
24 (n=164)	136.99 (135.81-138.17)	32.13 (31.01-33.25)	3.582* (2.68-4.08)	2.42* (1.75-3.08)
30 (n=149)	138.35 (137.22-139.45)	33.30 (32.21-34.39)	4.274* (3.46-5.08)	269* (2.01-3.17)
36 (n=165)	142.25 (140.87-143.63)	35.89 (34.57-37.21)	3.325* (2.42-4.22)	2.06* (1.38-2.74)
42 (n=148)	145.46 (143.90-147.02)	38.30 (37.92-38.67)	1.894 (1.00-2.78)	1.50 (0.78-2.22)
48 (n=160)	149.10 (147.6-150.6)	42.10 (40.59-43.61)	1.588 (0.68-2.48)	0.83 (0.41-1.25)

*p<0.05 with respect to basal value

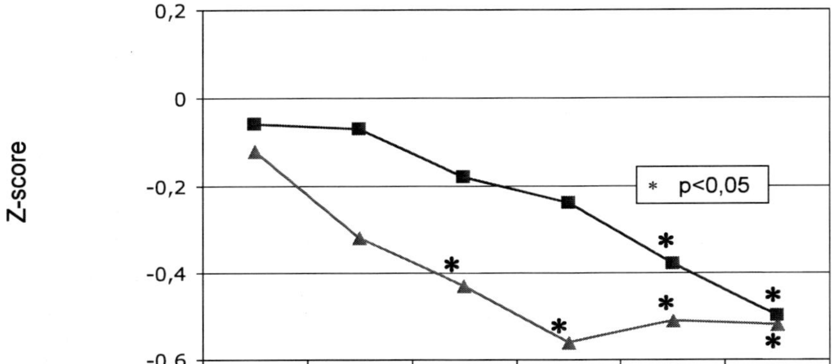

	Basal	6	12	18	24	30
Weight (Z-score)	-0,12	-0,32	-0,43	-0,56	-0,51	-0,52
Height (Z-score)	-0,06	-0,07	-0,18	-0,24	-0,38	-0,5

*p<0.05 with respect to basal value.

Figure 2. Changes in mean values of weight (z-score) and height (z-score) during 30 months (first stage).

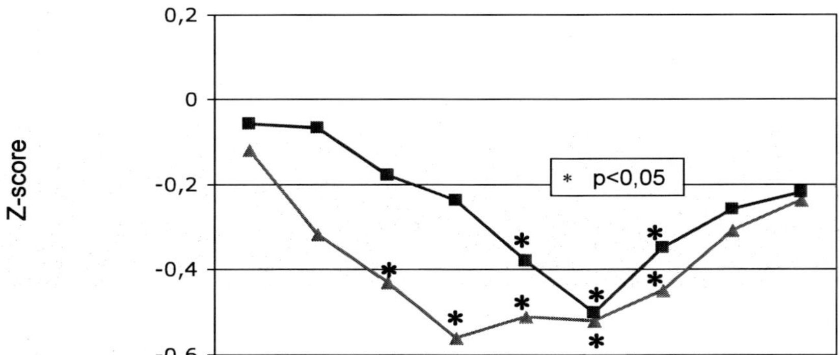

	Basal	6	12	18	24	30	36	42	48
Weight (Z-score)	-0,12	-0,32	-0,43	-0,56	-0,51	-0,52	-0,45	-0,31	-0,24
Height (Z-score)	-0,06	-0,07	-0,18	-0,24	-0,38	-0,5	-0,35	-0,26	-0,22

*p<0.05 with respect to basal value.

Figure 3. Changes in mean values of weight (z-score) and height (z-score) during 48 months (both stages).

At diagnosis, mean weight value in these patients was lower than mean weight expected for age in 0.697 kg (weight deficit). This difference increased to 4.274 kg after 30 months of treatment (first stage), even though it reduced later and was 1.588 kg after 48 months of treatment (second stage). In the same way, mean value of height was lower than expected mean height for age in 0.42 cm (height deficit) at diagnosis. This difference extended to 2.69 cm after 30 months (first stage), but it subsequently reduced and was 0.83 cm after 48 months of treatment (second stage). There were not any significant differences regarding sex, age at diagnosis or clinical subtype. There were no correlation between OROS-MPH dose and weight deficit and height deficit in every follow-up control. Figure 2 and 3 show the evolution of mean values of weight (z-score) and height (z-score) along 30 months after diagnosis (first stage) and 48 months after treatment (second stage), respectively. Basal value for weight (z-score) gradually decreased during the treatment, getting to significantly lower values ($p<0.05$) than basal value after 12 months. They kept low until 36 months of follow-up and subsequently recovered. Basal value of height (z-score) also decreased gradually during treatment, getting to significantly lower values ($p<0.05$) with respect to basal value after 24, 30 and 36 months, and subsequently recovered.

DISCUSSION

ADHD constitutes a potential issue of concern in health care with a relative significance attending its negative impact on the quality of life of the patient and the home environment. In addition, many adolescents will remain having problems in adult life, which bears a series of labor, social, economic and sanitary consequences [28, 29]. There is not any psychological and/or biological marker for this pathology, and diagnosis is based only upon clinical criteria [21, 24]. Stimulant drugs, and specifically MPH in our country, are the first line treatment in those patients diagnosed with ADHD [4-8], being this fact supported by many clinical trials that confirm the sustained efficacy of MPH in attention and behavioral symptoms, which allows, to a large extent, to optimize their familiar, academic and social situation [9,11,13,30]. Nevertheless, there seems to be a general concern about a virtual negative effect on height and weight growth. Regarding epidemiological aspects in this series, we should highlight that age corresponding at diagnosis displays a normal distribution with maximum incidence during school age, as well as a slight predominance of male sex (male/female ratio: 2.2) and the combined subtype; this data fits the results reported in the references [2,31-33]. These peculiarities allowed considering that the random sample was representative of a standard population of patients with ADHD and, therefore, there was not any reason to think about any statistical bias in the results and/or conclusions.

The conditio sine qua non to be included in this study was the prescription of OROS-MPH as a stimulant drug, since that was the only sustained-release preparation available in our country for a long enough time to complete an adequate follow up. In addition, the advantages of its pharmacokinetic profile make it preferable to the immediate release preparation [4-8], therefore being the stimulant drug of choice at that moment. Even though the request for complementary studies is not considered mandatory, the different entities to be considered in differential diagnosis of ADHD [34], justify, to a great extent, the blood, genetic, neurophysiological and neuroimaging studies accomplished in this group of patients, whose results show agenesis of corpus callosum as the only finding to be cited. The prescription in these patients was conditioned by the presentation of commercialized OROS-MPH (18, 36 and 54 mg; 27 mg has been recently added) and, especially by the necessary adjustment of dose depending on clinical response [35]. The total daily mean dose was increased systematically throughout the follow up in a similar way as previous studies did [6, 10, 13, 15, 18, 36, 37]. We did not prescribe doses of OROS-MPH that could virtually affect growth [22] (maximum dose was 1.81 mg/kg/day) and, so, always within the margin of safety and tolerability".

Absolute values for mean weight and height in these patients slightly increased (14.9 kg and 19.8 cm, respectively) along the period of treatment. Anyway, as this period passed, the differences with respect to expected values for age, in weight (weight deficit), as well as in height (height deficit), increased gradually, getting to top difference values after 30 months of treatment (4274 kg and 2.69 cm, respectively). When considering that initial weight and height were lower than expected for age, we could considerer that a weight deficit of 3.58 kg (1.43 kg/year) and a height deficit of 2.27 cm (0.91 cm/year) had accumulated. Nevertheless, beyond 36 months of treatment, and right after nutrition intervention, a progressive recovery of anthropometric variables was detected.

Accumulated weight and height deficit were not significant after 48 months of treatment, being 0.89 kg (0.22 kg/year) and 0.41 cm (0.1 cm/year), respectively. This evolutionary behavior of anthropometric variables in this group of patients leads to some considerations. On one side, the short-term observed weight and height deficit seemed to confirm the hypothesis of the negative effect of MPH on the growth of these patients [16-18,20- -23,25,38], which would demand us to introduce systematic registration of anthropometric variables as a mandatory procedure, as clinical guidelines and international consensus suggest [5-9]. On the other side, the medium-term recovery of anthropometric variables appears to confirm the hypothesis of *growth rebound*; that is, the effects of stimulant drugs, and specifically MPH, on the growth curve, would be a transitory condition that lessens as time passes by [18, 19, 24, 39-41].

Even though these two hypotheses may seem antagonistic, our data suggest that they could be complementary. Most previous studies on security and tolerability of MPH refer to a synchronous effect of this drug on weight and height [18, 23, 24, 37], and few references point at nutrition deficit as a mechanism potentially related to the growth retardation that these patients may show during treatment with MPH [22, 42]. A lack of temporal coincidence in this series among slow weight and height gain, which recalls the classical concept that a nutritional deficiency (acute malnutrition) initially manifests as a weight loss and implies growth retardation when maintained for a long period of time (chronic malnutrition).

This way, the growth rate would get to normality after body weight recovery. This means, data suggest that the anorexigenic effect of MPH would be the direct cause of the flattening in weight curve in these patients, whose maximum effects are observed between 18 and 30 months after the beginning of the treatment. Therefore, this sustained nutritional deprivation would be the main cause of proved growth retardation. The weight recovery would take place later, possibly in relation to dietary changes by families and/or pediatricians of these patients so as to offset the nutritional aggravation along the treatment with MPH. This could explain, to a great extent, the growth rebound in these patients.

This study presents several methodological limitations. First of all, a control group has not been included because of ethical implications, and, so, the results of weight, height and nutritional status of the patients have been compared to infant growth curves and charts which, on the other hand, are generally used as reference patterns in daily clinical practice. Setting up a control group of patients with mild to moderate ADHD and receiving no pharmacological treatment was not possible, since the total number of patients in these circumstances who were followed was rather limited, and many of them finally required MPH owing to progressive psycho-social and/or educational deterioration, and the rest faced diagnostic uncertainty. Second, we might have dispensed with the extreme age groups (preschool and adolescent groups) in order to avoid auxological variability. However, those groups were not excluded since the percentage of patients in these age bracket was small and their inclusion permitted the study to present an overall perspective of patients with ADHD.

In summary, the observed relationship between nutritional status and the negative effects on the weight and height curve in those patients under sustained treatment with OROS-MPH would require a nutritional optimization, as well as the introduction of pharmacological strategies (drug holidays) so as to return anthropometric variables to normal levels. Hence, the need to provide, simultaneously with multidisciplinary treatment, nutritional education programs to the patients and/or their families should be considered, in order to avoid the nutritional problems and the consequences that might be due to the treatment with MPH.

CONCLUSION

1. Maintained treatment with OROS-MPH at safe and tolerable doses has a negative effect on growth curve. After 30 months of treatment, accumulated weight and height deficit were 1.43 kg/year and 0.91 kg/year, respectively.
2. This negative effect initially manifests as a weight slowdown, being significant after 6 months of treatment. If this effect maintains, it carries a height slowdown, which is significant beyond 24 months of treatment.
3. The implementation of strategies of nutritional optimization in these patients allows the normalization of anthropometric variables (weight and height recovery). After 48 months of treatment (18 months after the beginning of nutrition intervention), accumulated weight and height deficit have reduced to 0.22 kg/year and 0.1 cm/year, respectively.
4. A systematic registration of anthropometric variables (weight and height) should be mandatory in every patient susceptible of treatment with OROS-MPH, and methodically compared with appropriate reference patterns.
5. Finally, the need of providing nutrition education programs to patients and/or their families, simultaneously with multimodal treatment, should be considered in order to counteract nutritional problems and their consequences due to treatment with OROS-MPH.

REFERENCES

[1] Cardo E, Servera M, Llobera J. Estimation of the prevalence of attention deficit hyperactivity disorder among the standard population on the island of Majorca. *Rev. Neurol.* 2007; 44: 10-14.

[2] Froelich TE, Lanphear BP, Epstein JN, Barbaresi WJ, Katusic SK, Kahn RS. Prevalence, recognition, and treatment of attention-deficit/hyperactivity disorder in a national sample of US children. *Arch. Pediatr. Adolesc. Med.* 2007; 161: 857-864.

[3] Merikangas KR, He JP, Brody D, Fisher PW, Bourdon K, Koretz DS. Prevalence and treatment of mental disorders among US children in the 2001-2004 NHANES. *Pediatrics.* 2010; 125: 75-81.

[4] American Academy of Pediatrics. Clinical practice guideline: diagnosis and evaluation of the child with attention-deficit/hyperactivity disorder. *Pediatrics.* 2000; 105: 1158-1170.

[5] American Academy of Child and Adolescent Psychiatry. Practice parameter for the use of stimulant medications in the treatment of children, adolescents, and adults. *J. Am. Acad. Child. Adolesc. Psychiatry.* 2002; 41(suppl 2): S26-S49.

[6] Kutcher S, Aman M, Brooks SJ, et al. International consensus statement on attention-deficit/hyperactivity disorder (ADHD) and disruptive behaviour disorders (DBDs): clinical implications and treatment practice suggestions. *European Neuropsychopharmacology.* 2004; 14:11-28.

[7] Rappley MD. Attention deficit-hyperactivity disorder. *N. Engl. J. Med.* 2005; 352: 165-173.

[8] National Institute for Health and Clinical Excellence (NICE). NICE clinical guideline 72: *attention-deficit/hyperactivity disorder* (ADHD). London, England: NICE; 2008.

[9] Pliszka S. AACAP Work Group on Quality Issues. Practice parameter for the assessment and treatment of children and adolescents with attention-deficit/hyperactivity disorder. *J. Am. Acad. Child. Adolesc. Psychiatry.* 2007; 46: 894-921.

[10] Wilens T, McBurnett K, Stein M, Lerner M, Spencer T, Wolraich M. ADHD treatment with once-daily OROS methylphenidate: final results from a long-term open-label study. *J. Am. Acad. Child. Adolesc. Psychiatry.* 2005; 44: 1015-1023.

[11] Brown RT, Amler RW, Freeman WS, et al. American Academy of Pediatrics, Committee on Quality Improvement, Subcommittee on Attention-Deficit/Hyperactivity Disorder. Treatment of attention-

deficit/hyperactivity disorder: overview of the evidence. *Pediatrics.* 2005; 115: e749-e757.

[12] Molina BS, Hinshaw SP, Swanson JM, et al. MTA Cooperative Group. The MTA at 8 years: prospective follow-up of children treated for combined-type ADHD in a multisite study. *J. Am. Acad. Child. Adolesc. Psychiatry.* 2009; 48: 484-500.

[13] Wolraich ML, Greenhill LL, Pelham W, et al. Randomized, controlled trial of OROS methylphenidate once a day in children with attention-deficit/hyperactivity disorder. *Pediatrics.* 2001; 108: 883-892.

[14] Mulas F, Roselló B, Morant A, Hernández S, Pitarch I. The effects of psychostimulants on the cognitive results and behaviour of children with the combined subtype of attention deficit with hyperactivity. *Rev. Neurol.* 2002; 35: 17-24.

[15] Fernández-Jaén A, Fernández-Mayoralas D, Calleja-Pérez B, Muñoz-Jareño N. Sustained effectiveness of osmotic-release methylphenidate: a study of 266 cases. *Rev. Neurol.* 2009; 48: 339-345.

[16] Poulton A, Cowell CT. Slowing of growth in height and weight on stimulants: A characteristic pattern. *J. Paediatr. Child. Health.* 2003; 39: 180-185.

[17] Lisska MC, Rivkees SA. Daily methylphenidate use slows the growth of children in a community sample. *J. Pediatr. Endocrinol. Metab.* 2003; 16: 711-718.

[18] MTA Cooperative Group. National Institute of Mental Health Multimodal Treatment Study of ADHD follow-up: changes in effectiveness and growth after the end of treatment. *Pediatrics.* 2004; 113:762-769.

[19] Spencer TJ, Faraone SV, Biederman J, Lerner M, Cooper KM, Zimmerman B. on behalf of the Concerta Study Group. Does prolonged therapy with a long-acting stimulant suppress growth in children with ADHD? *J. Am. Acad. Child. Adolesc. Psychiatry.* 2006; 45: 527-537.

[20] Pliszka S, Matthews TL, Braslow KJ, Watson MA. Comparative effects of methylphenidate and mixed salts amphetamine on height and weight in children with attention deficit hyperactivity disorder (ADHD). *J. Am. Acad. Child. Adolesc. Psychiatry.* 2006; 45: 520-527.

[21] Swanson JM, Greenhill LL, Wigal T, et al. Stimulant-related reduction of growth rates in the preschool ADHD treatment study PATS. *J. Am. Acad. Child. Adolesc. Psychiatry.* 2006; 45: 1304-1313.

[22] Charach A, Figueroa M, Chen S, Ickowics A, Schachar R. Stimulant treatment over 5 years: effects on growth. *J. Am. Acad. Child. Adolesc. Psychiatry*. 2006; 45: 415-421.

[23] Swanson JM, Elliott GR, Greenhill LL, et al. Effects of stimulant medication on growth rates across 3 years in the MTA follow-up. *J. Am. Acad. Child. Adolesc. Psychiatry*. 2007; 46: 1015-1027.

[24] Faraone SV, Biederman J, Morley CP, Spencer TC. Effect of stimulants on height and weight: a review of the literature. *J. Am. Acad. Child. Adolesc. Psychiatry*. 2008; 47: 994-1009.

[25] Zhang H, Du M, Zhuang S. Impact of long-term treatment of methylphenidate on height and weight of school age children with ADHD. *Neuropediatrics*. 2010; 41: 55-59.

[26] Caron M. Growth in the dopamine transporter knockout animal model of ADHD. *Neuropsychopharmacology*. 2004; 29(suppl 1):S55.

[27] Volkow ND, Wang GJ, Fowler JS. Relationship between blockade of dopamine transporters by oral methylphenidate and the increases in extracellular dopamine: therapeutic implications. *Synapse*. 2002; 43: 181-187.

[28] American Psychological Association. In: *Diagnostic and Statistical Manual of Mental Disorders*. 4th ed. Washington, DC: American Psychological Association; 2000.

[29] World Health Organization (WHO). *The Tenth Revision of the International Classification of Diseases and Related Health Problems*. Geneva, Switzerland: WHO; 1992.

[30] Swanson J, Gupta S, Williams L, Agler D, Lerner M, Wigal S. Efficacy of a new pattern of delivery of methylphenidate for the treatment of ADHD: effects on activity level in the classroom and on the playground. *J. Am. Acad. Child. Adolesc. Psychiatry*. 2002; 41: 1306-1314.

[31] Greenhill LL. Diagnosing attention-deficit/hyperactivity disorder in children. *J. Clin. Psychiatry*. 1998; 59(suppl 7): 31-41.

[32] Brown RT, Freeman WS, Perrin JM, et al. Prevalence and assessment of attention-deficit/hyperactivity disorder in primary care settings. *Pediatrics*. 2001; 107: e43.

[33] Cardo E, Severa-Barceló M. The prevalence of attention deficit hyperactivity disorder. *Rev. Neurol.* 2005; 40(suppl 1): S11-S15.

[34] Fernández M, Hidalgo I, Lora A, Sánchez L, Rodríguez L, Eddy LS, et al. La atención primaria y el trastorno por déficit de atención con/sin hiperactividad (TDAH). *Consenso multidisciplinar y evidencias para la puesta en práctica*. Madrid: ACINDES; 2009.

[35] Stein MA, Sarampote CS, Waldman ID, et al. A doseresponse study of OROS methylphenidate in children with attention-deficit/hyperactivity disorder. *Pediatrics.* 2003; 112: e404-e413.

[36] Wilens TE, McBurnett K, Bukstein O, et al. Multisite controlled study of OROS methylphenidate in the treatment of adolescents with attention-deficit/hyperactivity disorder. *Arch. Pediatr. Adolesc. Med.* 2006; 160: 82-90.

[37] Holtkamp K, Konrad K, Muller B, et al. Overweight and obesity in children with attention deficit/hyperactivity disorder. *Int. J. Obes. Relat. Metab. Disord.* 2004; 28: 685-689.

[38] Poulton A. Growth on stimulant medication; clarifying the confusion: a review. *Arch. Dis. Child.* 2005; 90: 801-806.

[39] Biederman J, Spencer TJ, Monuteaux MC, Faraone SV. A naturalistic 10-year prospective study of height and weight in children with attention-deficit hyperactivity disorder grown up: sex and treatment effects. *J. Pediatr.* 2010; 157: 635-640.

[40] Kramer JR, Loney J, Ponto LB, Roberts MA, Grossman S. Predictors of adult height and weight in boys treated with methylphenidate for childhood behaviour problems. *J. Am. Acad. Child. Adolesc. Psychiatry.* 2000; 39: 517-524.

[41] Dubnov-Raz G, Perry A, Berger I. Body mass index of children with attention-deficit/hyperactivity disorder. *J. Child. Neurol.* 2011; 26: 302-308.

[42] Charach A, Ickowicz A, Schachar R. Stimulant treatment over five years: adherence, effectiveness, and adverse effects. *J. Am. Acad. Child. Adolesc. Psychiatry.* 2004; 43:559-567.

In: ADHD ISBN: 978-1-62417-107-9
Editors: R. Thompson and N. J. Miller

Chapter 6

The Relation between Sluggish Cognitive Tempo and ADHD: A Critical Review

Maria Skounti
Department of Social Medicine,
University of Crete, Greece

Abstract

Sluggish Cognitive Tempo (SCT) is a cluster of symptoms including drowsiness, daydreaming, physical hypoactivity, lethargy and apathy. The SCT emerged in association with the ADHD-Inattentive (ADHD-I) type as a great percentage of children diagnosed within this subtype, also present SCT symptoms. Although items relevant to SCT were included in the DSM-IV field trials and were found to associate specifically with the inattentive type of ADHD, they were excluded from the final diagnostic criteria, because of their poor negative predictive power. This omission has led to a long- standing dispute regarding the validity of the ADHD-I type and the use of SCT symptoms as a discriminating factor for the ADHD subtypes. A related debate over the classification of the SCT construct has stimulated considerable research. Although, to date, the construct itself has not been adequately defined, many researchers have proposed that the SCT construct may represent a disorder that is a separate form, but highly co-morbid with ADHD. Additionally, it remains unclear, to what extent the SCT construct is clinically and diagnostically meaningful. The purpose of the present critical review is to analyze the complex relation between ADHD and SCT in terms of diagnostic classification, impairment and comorbidity and to provide future research directions.

Attention deficit hyperactivity disorder (ADHD) is among the most prevalent, heterogeneous and yet diagnostically controversial disorders of childhood (Skounti et al 2009). The conceptualization of ADHD has undergone significant change over the years, largely because of the dispute about the core deficits associated with the disorder (Baeyens et al 2006; Carlson and Mann 2002; Woo and Rey 2005).

Currently, the DSM-IV diagnostic criteria identify two dimensions of impairing symptoms, inattention and hyperactivity - impulsivity. Based on these symptoms dimensions, three subtypes of the disorder can be diagnosed: the predominantly inattentive (ADHD-I), the combined (ADHD-C) and the predominantly hyperactive- impulsive type (ADHD-HI) (AAP 2000; APA 1994).

These subtypes were defined in DSM-IV, mainly to reduce the heterogeneity of DSM-III-R AD/HD in terms of symptoms, impairment and demographics (Lahey et al 1994; Lahey and Willcutt 2010), but their validity is highly debating.

The most persisting debate in the ADHD classification history concerns the validity of the ADHD-I subtype. To date, there is a growing body of evidence suggesting that this subtype could be better conceptualized as a distinct disorder rather than as a related subtype of ADHD. (Adams et al 2008; Garner et al 2010; 2011; Milich et al. 2001; Penny et al 2009; Skansgaarde and Burns 1998).

Consistent with this approach, recent research suggests that the differences between the ADHD-I and ADHD-C types are not limited to the presence of hyperactive and impulsive symptoms, as these subtypes differ on several dimensions, such as social and academic impairment, age of onset, comorbidity, neuropsychological-cognitive processes and treatment response (Bauermeister et al 2011; Carlson and Mann 2002; Derefinko et al.2008). Therefore, it is possible that ADHD Inattentive symptoms index cognitive aspects of attention problems, while DSM-IV H/I symptoms may index behavioral aspects of a latent trait of the disorder, called disinhibition (Chhabildas et al. 2001; Garner et al 2011; Penny et al 2009; Solanto et al 2009).

Additionally, several studies indicate that the behavioral differences seen between the ADHD-I type and the other subtypes of the disorder may represent different types of attention problems and that the ADHD-C subtype is primarily associated with distractibility, while ADHD-I type is characterized by sluggish cognitive tempo (Chhabildas et al 2001; Derefinko et al 2008; Garner et al 2010; 2011; Harrington and Waldman 2010).

The concept of Sluggish Cognitve Tempo (SCT) is crucial and highly controversial in the ADHD classification. Sluggish cognitive tempo is a cluster of symptoms including drowsiness, daydreaming, physical hypoactivity, lethargy and apathy (Becker et al 2012; Garner et al 2011; Jacobson et al 2012; Skirbekk et al 2011).

The SCT emerged in association with ADHD-I type as a great percentage of children diagnosed within this subtype, also present SCT symptoms (Carlson and Mann 2002; Garner et al 2011; McBurnett et al 2001). Although items relevant to SCT were included in the DSM-IV field trials and were found to correlate specifically to the inattentive type of the disorder, they were excluded from the final diagnostic criteria, because of their poor negative predictive power (Carlson and Mann 2002; Hartman et al 2004; Harrington and Waldman 2010; Todd et al 2004). In other words, the absence of SCT symptoms did not predict the absence of ADHD-I type (Hinshaw 2001; McBurnett et al 2001; Todd et al 2004).

Basically, SCT items were eliminated as they failed to rule out the inattentive type that is associated with hyperactivity-impulsivity. The reasonable assertion that inattention unassociated with hyperactivity-impulsivity may be qualitatively different, was left aside (Hinsaw 2001).

To date there are many studies suggesting that SCT is not entirely explained by DSM-IV defined inattention (Jacobson et al 2012) and that current diagnostic criteria allow ADHD-I to be conceptualized as subthreshold ADHD-C or permit ADHD-I diagnosis in children with five or more H/I symptoms (Adams et al 2008; Hinsaw 2001; Milich et al. 2001; Schmitz et al 2010).

Obviously, this variability in diagnostic classification produces a heterogenous group of ADHD-I children and can explain the inconsistency existing among studies (Carlson and Mann 2001; McBurnett et al 2001; Milich et al. 2001).

For reducing the heterogeneity within the ADHD-I type, many researchers have proposed placing the ADHD-I type into a smaller category that is defined by only two or three hyperactive-impulsive symptoms (Adams et al 2008; Bauermeister et al 2011; Carr et al 2010; Derefinko et al 2008; Schmitz et al

2010), while others suggested the use of SCT symptoms as a marker for the ADHD-I type (Milich et al 2001; Schmitz et al 2010; Willcutt and Carlson 2005).

Evidence of both approaches is mixed. Using H/I symptoms as a diagnostic qualifier is conflicting, because the cutoff point to guide clinical decision making, remains understudied, subjective and developmental sensitive (Schmitz et al 2010).

On the other hand, using SCT as a discriminating factor for the ADHD subtypes is controversial because neither the construct itself has been adequately defined, nor the group it represents specified (Jacobson et al 2012; Penny et al 2009). Moreover, SCT symptoms are more severe in the ADHD-I type, but they are also present in the ADHD-C subtype and in other clinical conditions (Garner et al 2010; 2011; Harrington and Waldman 2010; Hartman et al 2004).

Little is also known about the relation between SCT symptoms and impairment. In their study, Carlson and Mann (2002) found that children with ADHD-I and high levels of SCT have greater social problems than children with ADHD-I and low levels of SCT. Contrary, SCT has been shown to be negatively associated with academic impairments (Becker et al 2012; Hartman et al. 2004; Mikami et al 2007).These results raise serious implications regarding the clinical utility of the SCT construct in diagnosis of ADHD.

What is especially challenging here, is the fact that the ADHD-I type is recorded in literature as less social and more academically impaired, while the ADHD-C type as equally impaired in both domains (Greatz et al 2001; Gaub and Carlson 1997; McBurnett et al. 1999; Mugnaini et al.2006; Montiel-Nava et al 2002; Skounti et al. 2010; Willcutt and Carlson 2005; Woo and Rey 2005). Thus, if the ADHD-I type with few or more SCT symptoms is not academically impaired, then the DSM-IV defined symptoms of inattention and not SCT are related with academic underachievement.

This assumption come in accordance with the results of the study of Wåhlstedt and Bohlin (2010), who have addressed the independent and interactive relations of DSM-IV defined inattention and SCT to academic achievement and found that only DSM-IV defined inattention symptoms were associated with academic impairments. Consistently, data from the study of Bauermeister et al (2011) indicated ADHD inattention as the primary determinant of impairment in ADHD.

Furthermore, common comorbid conditions related to all subtypes of ADHD and primary to the ADHD-I are internalizing problems, such as anxiety and mood disorders (Woo and Rey 2005). Interestingly, some studies support a positive association between SCT and internalizing problems (Hartman et al 2004). There is also some evidence that ADHD-I children with high levels of SCT symptoms are more withdrawn than children with moderate or none SCT symptoms (Carlson and Mann 2002; Mikami et al 2007).

Based on these associations, it can be assumed that either SCT is a separate condition reflecting internalizing problems comorbid with ADHD or that SCT is taping increased risk of subsequent development of co-occurrent mood and anxiety disorders. (Bauermeister et al.2011; Garner et al 2011; Harrington and Waldman 2010; Hartman et al 2004; Mikami et al 2007; Wåhlstedt and Bohlin 2010).

Oppositional Defiant Disorder (ODD) is one of the most common comorbid disorders related more to ADHD-C and HI type of the disorder and less with the Inattentive (Wåhlstedt and Bohlin 2010; Woo and Rey 2005). Although studies assessing the association of SCT and DSM-IV defined Inattention with ODD are almost nonexistent, there is some evidence suggesting that the presence of SCT behaviors may contribute to the lower level of ODD in ADHD-I type. It is also hypothesized that since ODD is strongly related to hyperactivity and impulsivity symptoms, that children with ADHD-I without SCT may have subthreshold ADHD-C type that make them vulnerable to ODD (Wåhlstedt and Bohlin 2010).

Undoubtedly, the field needs further research support in order to determine the extent to which SCT symptoms are associated with other conditions and functional impairment above and beyond the contribution of ADHD (Baeyens et al 2006; Bauermeister et al 2011; Becker et al 2012).

Conclusion- Clinical Implications

The SCT construct associated with ADHD has stimulated considerable research as current diagnostic criteria of ADHD-inattention cannot explain SCT symptoms. To date, neither the construct itself nor the group it represents are adequately defined.

SCT may constitute a subgroup of children with ADHD, but it may include children who do not fulfill DSM-IV criteria for ADHD. It is also possible that SCT symptoms are exhibited on a continuum and that are not specific to the ADHD-I subtype. This suggests that SCT symptoms may be quite common in children presenting with a variety of emotional and behavioral problems (Garner et al 2010; 2011; Jacobson et al 2012; Penny et al 2009).

The assessment of SCT symptoms above and beyond the ADHD diagnostic umbrella is clinically and diagnostically meaningful, because their presence indicates children who need further clinical evaluation and intervention. For incorporating though, SCT into the assessment scheme of ADHD an operational definition of SCT construct, valid measures and diagnostic decision rules are warrant.

Future studies assessing the independent and interactive relations of DSM-IV defined inattention and SCT to functional impairment are also extremely important. The relation between symptoms of a disorder and the consequent impairment is the most fundamental criterion to verify that the disorder is valid and warrants treatment (Chronis et al 2001).

Furthermore, the use of SCT as a marker for the ADHD-I type as suggested by many researchers, does not seem to create a more homogeneous subgroup that differs in terms of etiology, comorbidity and treatment response (Harrington and Waldman 2010).

To date there is no conclusive evidence that ADHD-I type shows a distinct pattern of neuropsychological features and impairment from that of ADHD-C type, even with limited SCT symptoms (Baeyens et al 2006; Chhabildas et al 2001; Willcutt and Carlson 2005; Woo and Rey 2005).

The issue here is not the subtype differentiation but the combination of available information to promote the most effective treatment (Derefinko et al 2008). Focusing more on a child's overall adjustment than on syndrome itself may promote more relevant diagnosis and effective management (Gordon et al 2006).

As traditional treatments seem to be less efficacious in treating the primary symptoms of the ADHD-I type, further research is needed to determine whether interventions designed to directly address the inattentive and SCT performance would be more effective than those applied for the ADHD-C type (Derefinko et al 2008; Solanto et al 2009).

In summary, by reviewing the available literature, although inadequate enough, the conclusion that seems to be reasonable is that the ADHD-I type and SCT are separate conditions highly correlated with common impairment features.

REFERENCES

Adams ZW, Derefinko KJ, Milich R, Fillmore MT. Inhibitory functioning across ADHD subtypes: Recent findings, clinical implications and future directions. *Dev. Disabil. Res. Rev.* 2008; 14(4):268-75.

American Academy of Pediatrics. Clinical practice guideline: diagnosis and evaluation of the child with attention-deficit/hyperactivity disorder. *Pediatrics* 2000; 105: 1158-1170.

American Psychiatric Association. The Diagnostic and Statistical Manual of Psychiatric Disorders. 4th ed. Washington, DC: American Psychiatric Association, 1994.

Baeyens D, Roeyers H, Walle JV. Subtypes of attention-deficit/hyperactivity disorder (ADHD): distinct or related disorders across measurement levels? *Child Psychiatry Hum. Dev.* 2006; 36(4):403-17.

Bauermeister JJ, Barkley RA, Bauermeister JA, Martínez JV, McBurnett K. Validity of the sluggish cognitive tempo, inattention, and hyperactivity symptom dimensions: neuropsychological and psychosocial correlates. *J. Abnorm. Child Psychol.* 2012; 40(5): 683-97.

Becker SP, Langberg JM. Sluggish cognitive tempo among young adolescents with ADHD: Relations to mental health, academic, and social Functioning. *J. Atten. Disord.* 2012 Mar 21. [DOI: 10.1177/1087054711 435411]

Carlson CL, Mann M. Sluggish cognitive tempo predicts a different pattern of impairment in the attention deficit hyperactivity disorder, predominantly inattentive type. *J. Clin. Child Adolesc. Psychol.* 2002; 31(1):123-9.

Chhabildas N, Pennington BF, Willcutt EG. A comparison of the neuropsychological profiles of the DSM-IV subtypes of ADHD. *J. Abnorm. Child Psychol.* 2001;29(6):529-40.

Chronis AM, Fabiano GA, Gnagy EM,Wymbs BT, Burrows-MacLean L, Pelham W. Comprehensive, sustained behavioral and pharmacological treatment for attention- deficit/ hyperactivity disorder: A case study. *Cognitive and Behavioral Practice* 2001;8: 346-359.

Derefinko KJ, Adams ZW, Milich R, Fillmore MT, Lorch EP, Lynam DR. Response style differences in the inattentive and combined subtypes of attention-deficit/hyperactivity disorder. *J. Abnorm. Child Psychol.* 2008;36(5):745-58.

Garner AA, Marceaux JC, Mrug S, Patterson C, Hodgens B. Dimensions and correlates of attention deficit/hyperactivity disorder and Sluggish Cognitive Tempo. *J. Abnorm. Child Psychol.* 2010; 38(8):1097-107.

Garner AA, Marceaux JC, Mrug S, Patterson C, Hodgens B. Dimensions and correlates of attention deficit/hyperactivity disorder and Sluggish Cognitive Tempo. *J. Abnorm. Child Psychol.* 2010; 38(8):1097-107.

Gaub M, Carlson C. Behavioral characteristics of DSM-IV ADHD subtypes in a school-based population. *J. Abnorm. Child Psychol.* 1997; 25: 103-111.

Gordon M, Antshel K, Faraone S, Barkley R, Lewandowski L, Hudziak JJ, Biederman J, Cunningham C. Symptoms versus impairment: the case for respecting DSM-IV's Criterion D. *J. Atten. Disord.* 2006; 9 (3):465-75.

Graetz BW, Sawyer MG, Hazell PL, Arney F, Baghurst P. Validity of DSM-IV ADHD subtypes in a nationally representative sample of Australian children and adolescents. *J. Am. Acad. Child Adolesc. Psychiatry* 2001; 40(12): 1410-7.

Harrington KM, Waldman ID. Evaluating the utility of sluggish cognitive tempo in discriminating among DSM-IV ADHD subtypes. *J. Abnorm. Child Psychol.* 2010; 38(2): 173-84.

Hartman CA, Willcutt EG, Rhee SH, Pennington BF. The relation between sluggish cognitive tempo and DSM-IV ADHD. *J. Abnorm. Child Psychol.* 2004; 32(5):491-503.

Hinshaw SP. Is the Inattentive type of ADHD a separate disorder? *Clinical Psychology: Science and Practice* 2001; 8(4)498-501.

Jacobson LA, Murphy-Bowman SC, Pritchard AE, Tart-Zelvin A, Zabel TA, Mahone EM. Factor Structure of a Sluggish Cognitive Tempo Scale in Clinically-Referred Children. *J. Abnorm. Child Psychol.* 2012 May 8. [DOI:10.1007/s10802-012-9643-6]

Lahey BB, Applegate B, McBurnett K, Biederman J, Greenhill L, Hynd GW, Barkley RA et al. DSM-IV field trials for attention deficit hyperactivity disorder in children and adolescents. *Am. J. Psychiatry* 1994; 151(11):1673-85.

Lahey BB, Willcutt EG. Predictive validity of a continuous alternative to nominal subtypes of attention-deficit/hyperactivity disorder for DSM-V. *J. Clin. Child Adolesc. Psychol.* 2010; 39(6):761-75.

McBurnett K, Pfiffner LJ, Frick PJ. Symptom properties as a function of ADHD type: an argument for continued study of sluggish cognitive tempo. *J. Abnorm. Child Psychol.* 2001;29(3):207-13.

McBurnett K, Pfiffner LJ, Willcutt E, Tamm L, Lerner M, Ottolini YL, Furman MB. Experimental cross-validation of DSM-IV types of attention-deficit/hyperactivity disorder. *J. Am. Acad. Child Adolesc. Psychiatry* 1999; 38(1):17-24.

Mikami AY, Huang-Pollock CL, Pfiffner LJ, McBurnett K, Hangai D. Social skills differences among attention-deficit/hyperactivity disorder types in a chat room assessment task. *J. Abnorm. Child Psychol.* 2007; 35(4):509-21.

Milich R, Balentine AC, Lynam DR. ADHD Combined Type and ADHD Predominantly Inattentive Type Are Distinct and Unrelated Disorders. *Clinical Psychology: Science and Practice* 2001; 8: 463–488.

Montiel-Nava C, Pena JA, Lopez M, Salas M, Zurga JR, Montiel-Barbero I, Pirela D, Cardozo JJ. Estimations of the prevalence of attention deficit hyperactivity disorder in Marabino children. *Rev. Neurol.* 2002; 35: 1019-24. [In Spanish]

Mugnaini D, Masi G, Brovedani P, Chelazzi C, Marzenka M, Romagnoli C, Zuddas A. Teacher reports of ADHD symptoms in Italian children at the end of first grade. *European Psychiatry* 2006; 21(6):419-426.

Penny AM, Waschbusch DA, Klein RM, Corkum P, Eskes G. Developing a measure of sluggish cognitive tempo for children: content validity, factor structure, and reliability. *Psychol. Assess* 2009;21(3):380-9.

Schmitz M, Ludwig H, Rohde LA. Do hyperactive symptoms matter in ADHD-I restricted phenotype? *J. Clin. Child Adolesc. Psychol.* 2010; 39(6):741-8.

Skansgaard EP, Burns GL. Comparison of DSM-IV ADHD combined and predominantly inattention types: Correspondence between teacher ratings and direct observations of Innatentive,hyperactivity/impulsivity,slow cognitive tempo, oppositional defiant,and overt conduct disorder symptoms. *Child and Family Behavior therapy* 1998; 20(1):2-14.

Skirbekk B, Hansen BH, Oerbeck B, Kristensen H. The relationship between sluggish cognitive tempo, subtypes of attention-deficit/hyperactivity disorder, and anxiety disorders. *J. Abnorm. Child Psychol.* 2011; 39(4):513-25.

Skounti M, Giannoukas S, Dimitriou E, Nikolopoulou S, Linardakis E, Philalithis A. Prevalence of attention deficit hyperactivity disorder in schoolchildren in Athens. Social and academic impairment. *ADHD Atten. Def. Hyp. Disord.* 2010; 2(3):127-132.

Skounti M, Mpitzaraki K, Philalithis A, Galanakis E. Clinical evaluation of children testing positive in screening tests for attention deficit/hyperactivity disorder: A preliminary report. *Eur. J. Psych.* 2009; 23: 115-120.

Solanto MV, Pope-Boyd SA, Tryon WW, Stepak B. Social functioning in predominantly inattentive and combined subtypes of children with ADHD. *J. Atten. Disord.* 2009; 13(1):27-35.

Todd RD, Rasmussen ER, Wood C, Levy F, Hay DA. Should sluggish cognitive tempo symptoms be included in the diagnosis of attention-deficit/hyperactivity disorder? *J. Am. Acad. Child Adolesc. Psychiatry* 2004; 43(5):588-97.

Wåhlstedt C, Bohlin G. DSM-IV-defined inattention and sluggish cognitive tempo: independent and interactive relations to neuropsychological factors and comorbidity. *Child Neuropsychol.* 2010; 16(4):350-65.

Willcutt EG, Carlson CL. The diagnostic validity of attention deficit /hyperactivity disorder. *Clinical Neuroscience Research* 2005; 5:219-232.

Woo BS, Rey JM. The validity of the DSM-IV subtypes of attention-deficit/ hyperactivity disorder. *Aust. N. Z. J. Psychiatry* 2005; 39(5):344-53.

INDEX

A

academic performance, 10, 24
access, 25, 26, 78
acid, 16, 96
activity level, 10, 67, 119
adaptation, 99
adjustment, 32, 100, 114, 126
adolescents, 32, 44, 62, 63, 64, 76, 77, 78, 79, 96, 98, 113, 117, 120, 127, 128
Adult Attachment Interview, 35, 39, 59
adulthood, 8, 9, 59, 62
adults, 3, 8, 9, 11, 17, 22, 30, 31, 33, 62, 78, 101, 117
adverse effects, 120
advertisements, 8
aetiology, 36, 62, 65, 67
age, 3, 6, 40, 45, 62, 64, 83, 86, 98, 106, 108, 109, 110, 111, 112, 113, 114, 115, 119, 122
aggression, 58
alcohol abuse, 32
alertness, 17
American Psychiatric Association (APA), 2, 8, 10, 30, 60, 62, 66, 76, 122, 127
American Psychological Association, 66, 98, 119
amphetamines, 15, 19
anger, 36, 46, 47, 51, 54
antagonism, 49
anxiety, 3, 6, 18, 44, 69, 124, 125, 129
anxiety disorder, 6, 125, 129
apathy, 121, 123
appetite, 19
arousal, 37
assessment, 12, 63, 64, 65, 75, 77, 84, 117, 119, 126, 129
asthma, 73
attachment, 35, 36, 37, 38, 39, 40, 41, 42, 49, 58, 59, 60
attachment theory, 37, 40, 58
attitudes, 39, 65, 66, 67, 73, 74, 75, 77, 78, 79
authority, 52
awareness, 8, 9, 10, 50

B

barriers, 30, 74
basal ganglia, 95
base, 12, 22, 58, 67
behavioral problems, 125
behaviors, 125
beneficial effect, 26
benefits, 2, 5, 10, 20, 23, 28, 76
bias, 114
biochemistry, 108
biofeedback, 70
biological markers, 95
blame, 14, 42, 43, 51

blood, 3, 18, 108, 109, 114
body mass index (BMI), 106, 108, 109, 110
body weight, 115
borderline personality disorder, 48, 51
brain, 14, 15, 17, 18, 28, 69, 82, 83, 95, 96, 98, 99, 101, 102
brain damage, 69
brain functions, 15, 17
breathing, 57
bulimia, 66
bulimia nervosa, 66

C

calorie, 108
campaigns, 8, 9
caregivers, 63
case study, 35, 38, 127
casting, 47
causation, 48
central nervous system (CNS), 2, 17, 32
cerebellum, 95, 96
cerebral palsy, 83
cerebrum, 95
chemical(s), 17, 18, 28, 69
child development, 32
childhood, 3, 7, 9, 50, 59, 73, 99, 120, 122
children, 3, 8, 10, 11, 12, 13, 14, 19, 22, 27, 31, 32, 33, 36, 37, 39, 41, 44, 45, 51, 55, 56, 59, 60, 63, 64, 67, 70, 72, 75, 76, 77, 78, 81, 82, 83, 84, 85, 86, 87, 88, 89, 93, 94, 95, 96, 97, 98, 99, 100, 101, 117, 118, 119, 120, 121, 123, 124, 125, 126, 128, 129
chromosome, 97
clarity, 3
classes, 25
classification, 2, 36, 108, 121, 122, 123
classroom, 7, 9, 10, 19, 20, 63, 65, 67, 72, 82, 93, 98, 119
classroom teachers, 67
clients, 19, 66, 68, 73
clinical application, 58
clinical syndrome, 67, 68, 71
clinical trials, 113
clone, 50
closure, 47
clothing, 82
cognitive function, 17
cognitive process, 122
collaboration, ix, 61, 63, 64, 72, 85, 108
collagen, 97
common symptoms, 12
communication, 15, 38, 62, 63, 74
community, 9, 73, 75, 81, 82, 83, 89, 118
comorbidity, 81, 82, 83, 95, 96, 97, 105, 107, 122, 126, 130
complement, 50
complete blood count, 108
complexity, 37
complications, 69
computed tomography, 96
computer, 109
conceptualization, 122
concordance, 70
conduct disorder, 36, 60, 129
conflict, 37, 53, 98
consensus, 74, 76, 88, 115, 117
consent, 87
construction, 35, 40, 49, 69
consumption, 4, 67, 69, 76
control group, 115
controversial, 62, 77, 122, 123, 124
conversational analysis (CA), 35, 38, 40, 59, 128
conversations, 7, 21, 38, 42, 49
cooperation, 87
coordination, 74, 81, 82, 83, 85, 87, 89, 95, 97, 98, 99, 100, 101, 102
coping strategies, 24
corpus callosum, 109, 114
correlation, 109, 113
cortex, 96, 101
cost, 27, 72, 73, 75, 77
counseling, 11
cross-cultural comparison, 85
cross-validation, 128
cues, 29
culture, 32
cycles, 50

D

daily living, 82, 83, 89
deficiency, 115
deficit, 9, 30, 32, 33, 58, 59, 61, 62, 76, 77, 78, 79, 82, 100, 101, 102, 105, 106, 108, 111, 112, 114, 115, 116, 117, 118, 119, 120, 122, 127, 128, 129, 130
depressants, 1, 2, 4, 16, 17, 18, 32
depression, 62, 66, 69, 77
deprivation, 20, 115
destruction, 55
Developmental Coordination Disorder (DCD), ix, x, 81, 82, 83, 84, 85, 89, 90, 91, 93, 94, 95, 96, 97, 99, 100
developmental psychopathology, 60
Diagnostic and Statistical Manual of Mental Disorders, 63, 108, 119
diagnostic classification, 122, 123
diagnostic criteria, xi, 2, 6, 8, 89, 121, 122, 123, 125
Diagnostic Statistical Manual, 2
diet, 4, 11, 69, 70
differential diagnosis, 114
dinosaurs, 54
direct observation, 129
disability, 62, 64
discourse analysis, 35, 40
disorder, 3, 5, 6, 7, 8, 9, 12, 14, 21, 30, 31, 32, 33, 55, 58, 59, 61, 62, 68, 76, 77, 78, 79, 82, 83, 84, 96, 98, 99, 100, 101, 102, 105, 106, 117, 118, 119, 120, 121, 122, 123, 125, 126, 127, 128, 129, 130
disruptive behaviours, 19
dissociation, 59
distress, 42, 53
distribution, 5
doctors, 18, 19, 31
DOI, 127, 128
domestic violence, 36, 41, 60
dopamine, 1, 2, 15, 16, 17, 19, 96, 107, 119
dopaminergic, 17, 95, 97
dorsolateral prefrontal cortex, 95
dosage, 19, 20, 21, 22, 28
drawing, 82, 94
drug therapy, 5, 28, 29, 31, 105, 106
drugs, 1, 2, 4, 5, 9, 15, 17, 18, 19, 20, 21, 22, 24, 26, 27, 28, 29, 105, 107, 113, 115
DSM, 5, 8, 10, 108
DSM-IV-TR, 63, 98
dual task, 100

E

eating disorders, 60
education, 4, 11, 32, 62, 64, 67, 72, 78, 87, 106, 116
educational psychologists, 51
educational psychology, 68
electroencephalograph, 4, 11
elementary school, 86
emission, 96
emotionality, 13
encephalitis, 14
environment, 11, 18, 66, 68, 69, 70, 72, 113
environmental stress, 66
epidemic, 14, 36
ethical implications, 115
ethics, 87
etiology, 126
evidence, 12, 22, 37, 55, 61, 64, 74, 82, 95, 98, 118, 122, 125, 126
evolution, 31, 113
exaggeration, 9
examinations, 109
exclusion, 3, 53, 54
execution, 95
executive function, 15
exposure, 69

F

fairness, 44
false belief, 67
families, 39, 43, 44, 45, 46, 51, 58, 59, 62, 63, 70, 73, 115, 116
family environment, 37
family functioning, vii, 62
family life, 29, 44, 55

family members, 9, 11, 35, 37, 38, 39, 40, 44, 47, 74
family therapy, 38, 58
fatty acids, 70
feelings, 35, 39
female rat, 109, 113
field trials, 121, 123, 128
food, 67, 70
forensic services, 62
frontal lobe, 96
functional imaging, 95

G

GABA, 16, 96
general practitioner, 63, 69, 78
genes, 48, 50, 96, 97, 102
genetic factors, 37
genetic predisposition, 69
genetics, 14, 82, 83, 96, 98, 101
genome, x, 82, 96, 97, 102
glasses, 13
globus, 95
grades, 24
group work, 29
growth, 29, 105, 107, 108, 109, 113, 114, 115, 116, 118, 119
guidance, 63
guidelines, 61, 62, 63, 64, 65, 72, 74, 76, 78, 79, 115
guilt, 42
gymnastics, 82

H

hair, 50
handwriting, 83, 94, 97
headache, 19
health, 8, 22, 31, 32, 61, 62, 63, 68, 70, 72, 73, 74, 75, 76, 78, 94, 108, 113
health care, 31, 63, 108, 113
health services, 62, 64, 73, 74, 75
height, 106, 107, 108, 109, 110, 111, 112, 113, 114, 115, 116, 118, 119, 120
hemiplegia, 83
heredity, 14, 42, 53
heterogeneity, 97, 122, 123
high school, 86
higher education, 5
history, 2, 31, 49, 63, 122
homework, 21, 23
hyperactivity, 1, 5, 7, 8, 10, 11, 12, 14, 17, 28, 29, 30, 32, 33, 36, 61, 62, 72, 76, 77, 78, 79, 81, 82, 87, 89, 100, 101, 102, 105, 106, 108, 117, 118, 119, 120, 122, 123, 125, 127, 128, 129, 130
hyperactivity-impulsivity, 123
hyper-focused state, 1, 2, 4, 5, 22, 29
hypersensitivity, 66
hypothalamus, 107
hypothesis, 14, 17, 96, 114

I

ICE, 63
identification, 3, 30, 62
impairments, 93, 95, 97, 124
improvements, 10, 73
impulsive, 4, 5, 6, 17, 18, 28, 122, 123
impulsiveness, 14, 22, 85
impulsivity, 5, 7, 8, 10, 11, 12, 62, 72, 106, 108, 122, 123, 125, 129
in utero, 69
inattention, 5, 6, 10, 12, 17, 26, 28, 62, 72, 81, 87, 89, 106, 122, 123, 124, 125, 126, 127, 129, 130
incidence, 113
independence, 44, 45, 46
individuals, 1, 2, 3, 4, 5, 7, 8, 9, 10, 11, 12, 13, 14, 15, 16, 17, 18, 19, 20, 21, 22, 23, 24, 25, 26, 27, 28, 29, 30, 32, 38, 39, 62, 66
infancy, 58, 59
information sharing, 62
infrastructure, 74
inheritance, 49, 50, 51
inhibition, 14, 94, 96, 101
inhibitor, 95, 107
inner world, 37

insecurity, 56, 58
integration, 62, 94
intelligence, 54, 83
internalizing, 124, 125
International Classification of Diseases, 5, 119
intervention, 4, 11, 72, 73, 82, 94, 98, 100, 105, 106, 107, 108, 114, 116, 126
intervention strategies, 72
investment, 43
IQ scores, 25
irritability, 3, 18, 22
issues, 31, 75, 95

J

junior high school, 86, 87
juvenile delinquency, 66, 79

L

languages, 85
lead, 5, 6, 44, 56, 72, 82, 83, 97, 98
learners, 25
learning, 25, 32, 33, 62, 95, 100
learning process, 95
legs, 102
leisure, 7
lesions, 82, 95, 96
lethargy, 121, 123
light, 26, 73
Likert scale, 85
liver, 108
locus, 95, 97
loneliness, 56
loss of appetite, 3, 18, 20
lying, 13, 47

M

majority, 9, 25, 66, 73, 86
malnutrition, 115
management, 35, 62, 64, 66, 67, 68, 70, 71, 73, 74, 75, 76, 77, 78, 126
mapping, 101
marketing, 9
marriage, 55
masking, 29
mass, 106, 109, 120
measurement(s), 109, 127
medical, 48, 62, 63, 64, 65, 66, 68, 69, 71, 72, 73, 74, 76, 83, 93
medication, 1, 2, 3, 4, 5, 10, 11, 12, 14, 15, 18, 19, 20, 21, 22, 23, 24, 26, 27, 28, 29, 30, 32, 63, 64, 68, 70, 71, 72, 73, 75, 82, 94, 98, 101, 119, 120
medicine, 99
memory, 24, 95
mental disorder, 2, 76, 82, 98, 117
mental health, 31, 36, 62, 64, 65, 73, 74, 76, 78, 127
mental health professionals, 63, 64
mental retardation, 32, 83
mental state, 63
meta-analysis, 95
methodology, 68
methylphenidate, 4, 10, 15, 19, 20, 26, 32, 100, 101, 106, 107, 117, 118, 119, 120
middle class, 86
models, 36, 40
modification of ADHD symptoms, 1
mood disorder, 6, 124
morbidity, 63
motor control, 82, 83, 98, 99
motor skills, 94, 96, 99, 100
MRI, 95, 101
muscular dystrophy, 83

N

National Health Service (NHS), 40
National Institute of Mental Health, 78, 118
National Survey, 8
negative consequences, 23
negative effects, 4, 19, 22, 116
neglect, 2, 22
nervous system, 2, 32, 99
neuroimaging, 108, 109, 114
neurons, 15, 95, 97

neuroprotection, 97
neuropsychiatry, 68
neurotransmitter(s), 1, 15, 16, 19
neurotransmitter dopamine, 1, 15, 17
NHANES, 117
norepinephrine, 15, 17, 19, 95, 107
normal development, 44
normal distribution, 113
North America, 2, 5, 7
nursery school, 86
nutrition, 106, 107, 108, 114, 115, 116
nutritional status, 115, 116

O

obesity, 120
occipital lobe, 96
occupational therapy, 70, 94
oppositional behaviour, 7
Oppositional Defiant Disorder (ODD), 125
optimization, vii, x, xi, 106, 108, 116
organize, 15
osmotic release oral system methylphenidate (OROS-methylphenidate), 106, 107

P

parenting, 36, 39, 45, 65, 66, 69, 72
parents, 3, 9, 11, 13, 19, 36, 39, 41, 50, 51, 55, 63, 65, 67, 70, 73, 74, 76, 85, 86, 93, 98
participants, 17, 20, 24, 26, 68, 86, 87
pathophysiology, 84, 95
pediatrician, 108
percentile, 88, 89, 90, 91, 92
permit, 123
personal relations, 7
personality, 6, 42, 48, 50, 51, 52
pharmaceutical, 32
pharmacological treatment, 115, 127
pharmacotherapy, 64, 71, 78
phenotype, 97, 129
physical resemblance, 48
physical therapy, 94
physicians, 64, 76
pilot study, 69
placebo, 20, 24
playing, 7, 26, 82
poetry, 12
polymorphism, 97
poor performance, 83
population, 3, 22, 25, 31, 62, 66, 83, 93, 106, 114, 117, 128
post-traumatic stress disorder, 36
pregnancy, 62
preparation, 2, 95, 114
preschool, 64, 109, 115, 118
prescription drugs, 3, 22
prevention, 33
primary function, 15
primary school, 68, 69, 70, 71
principles, 25, 63
probe, 55
professionals, 6, 10, 11, 12, 23, 29, 37, 61, 62, 63, 64, 65, 66, 67, 68, 69, 70, 71, 72, 74, 75, 76
prognosis, 65, 83, 97
programming, 11
propaganda, 8
proposition, 38, 47
psychiatric disorders, 78
psychiatry, 31, 32, 63, 68
psychologist, 46, 64, 67, 75, 79
psychology, 31, 32, 63
psychometric properties, 85
psychopharmacology, 32, 33
psychostimulants, 118
psychotherapy, 11
publishing, 76

Q

quality of life, 94, 101, 113
questionnaire, 68, 71, 85, 86, 88, 93, 99

R

rating scale, 65, 69, 71, 85
reactions, 14, 16
reading, 71, 74
reality, 77
recognition, 63, 117
recommendations, 64, 65, 67, 72
recovery, 114, 115, 116
rehabilitation, 31
relevance, 3, 51
reliability, 85, 129
remission, 76
requirements, 26, 40
researchers, 8, 10, 17, 20, 24, 26, 27, 29, 121, 123, 126
resilience, 60
resolution, 48, 50, 77
resources, 19
response, x, 3, 44, 49, 54, 59, 70, 82, 107, 114, 122, 126
restless legs syndrome, 97
restrictions, 74
restructuring, 19
retardation, 83, 115
risk, 20, 22, 25, 88, 89, 92, 95, 97, 125
rules, 20, 126

S

sadness, 3, 18
safety, 55, 114
salts, 118
schizophrenia, 66, 77
school, 2, 5, 6, 9, 19, 20, 21, 22, 23, 24, 27, 31, 41, 53, 54, 56, 57, 62, 63, 64, 65, 67, 68, 69, 70, 72, 73, 76, 79, 81, 82, 83, 85, 86, 88, 89, 90, 91, 97, 108, 109, 113, 119, 128
scope, 24, 60
scripts, 39
SCT, 121, 123, 124, 125, 126
security, 115
sedative, 16
self-regulation, 11, 27
sensitivity, 17, 33, 93
sensors, 95
serum, 108
sex, 86, 108, 109, 110, 113, 120
sexually transmitted diseases, 62
shape, 37, 38
showing, 9, 17, 37
signals, 15, 17, 18
signs, 3, 13, 18
sleep deprivation, 20
SNP, 97
social behavior, 20, 23, 32
social environment, 16, 27, 28, 29, 57, 75, 125
social relationships, 22, 27, 29
social services, 41, 63, 78
social skills, 4, 11, 16, 21, 27, 28, 29, 30, 63, 72
social withdrawal, 20, 22, 23, 26, 27, 29, 30
social workers, 63, 64, 65, 66, 68
spatial learning, 32
special education, 67
specialists, 64, 66
speech, 70
spending, 26
stability, 94, 100
standard deviation, 109
state(s), 1, 2, 3, 4, 5, 22, 29, 41, 44, 56, 63, 98
stimulant, 1, 2, 3, 4, 5, 10, 11, 12, 14, 15, 16, 17, 18, 19, 22, 23, 24, 25, 26, 27, 28, 29, 30, 31, 33, 64, 71, 73, 101, 105, 107, 113, 114, 115, 117, 118, 119, 120
stimulation, 18, 96
stimulus, 16
stress, 37, 56, 57
striatum, 107
structure, 70, 129
style, 25, 58, 66, 69, 72, 127
succession, 51
susceptibility, 32
symptoms, 1, 2, 3, 4, 5, 6, 7, 8, 9, 10, 12, 13, 14, 15, 16, 17, 18, 20, 25, 27, 28, 29, 30, 62, 67, 71, 73, 76, 94, 95, 97, 100, 105,

107, 113, 121, 122, 123, 124, 125, 126, 129, 130
synapse, 15
syndrome, 82, 83, 84, 86, 88, 89, 90, 91, 92, 93, 97, 102, 126

T

target, 87
Task Force, 60
teacher support, 70
teachers, 3, 19, 63, 65, 67, 68, 69, 70, 71, 72, 75, 76, 77, 86, 98
team sports, 29
teams, 62, 73, 76
technetium, 96
techniques, 63
teens, 11
temperament, 52, 59
tempo, 123, 127, 128, 129, 130
temporal lobe, 96
tension(s), 42, 75
testing, 25, 65, 129
thalamus, 14
therapeutic approaches, 63
therapy, 2, 4, 5, 11, 16, 18, 23, 27, 28, 29, 30, 37, 63, 64, 67, 70, 74, 94, 105, 107, 118, 129
thyroid, 108
tones, 97
top-down, 40
training, 4, 11, 63, 65, 66, 70, 72
training programs, 63
traits, 49, 51
tranquilizers, 50
transcription, 39
transformation, 58
translation, 12, 85
transmission, 96
trauma, 41, 60
treatment, 3, 4, 6, 10, 11, 12, 14, 18, 28, 29, 30, 31, 33, 61, 62, 64, 65, 66, 67, 68, 69, 70, 71, 72, 73, 74, 75, 76, 77, 78, 84, 94, 101, 105, 106, 108, 109, 110, 111, 112, 113, 114, 115, 116, 117, 118, 119, 120, 122, 126
treatment methods, 4, 18
trial, 30, 78, 95, 100, 118
triangulation, ix, 36

U

underproduction, 15
unhappiness, 57
universities, 3

V

variables, x, xi, 73, 105, 106, 107, 108, 109, 114, 116
variations, 66
violence, 37, 56, 58, 60, 66
vitamins, 70

W

walking, 83
Washington, 60, 76, 98, 103, 119, 127
weight loss, 115
well-being, 28
Western countries, ix, 61
William James, 14
withdrawal, 20, 23, 27
work environment, 19
workers, 3, 19, 63, 78
workplace, 19, 27
World Health Organization (WHO), 85, 119

Y

young people, 36, 78